All About

Hip Replacement

A Patient's Guide

RICHARD TRAHAIR

Melbourne

OXFORD UNIVERSITY PRESS

Oxford   Auckland   New York

OXFORD UNIVERSITY PRESS AUSTRALIA
Oxford New York
Athens Auckland Bangkok Bogota Bombay
Buenos Aires Calcutta Cape Town Dar es Salaam
Delhi Florence Hong Kong Istanbul Karachi
Kuala Lumpur Madras Madrid Melbourne
Mexico City Nairobi Paris Port Moresby
Singapore Taipei Tokyo Toronto Warsaw
and associated companies in
Berlin Ibadan

OXFORD is a trade mark of Oxford University Press

National Library of Australia
Cataloguing-in-publication data:

Trahair, Richard C. S.
All about hip replacement: a patient's guide.

Bibliography.
Includes index.
ISBN 0 19 554112 X.

1. Total hip replacement – Popular works. I. Title.

617.581

Edited by Cathryn Game
Diagrams by Paul Lennon
Indexed by the author
Text and cover designed by Anitra Blackford
Typeset by Solo Typesetting
Printed through Bookpac Production Services, Singapore
Published by Oxford University Press
253 Normanby Road, South Melbourne, Australia

Preface

Osteoarthritis — or 'wear and tear' arthritis — is a very common condition, most often seen in elderly people, although also seen in younger people. The hip is the major joint in the lower limb that is most affected by osteoarthritis, and ultimately hip joint replacement might be the only cure. This surgical procedure, although first done more than a hundred years ago, was really pioneered by Sir John Charnley, a British surgeon, in the 1960s. Since then hip joint replacement has become the most common artificial joint procedure performed worldwide. It has brought pain relief and increased activity to millions of people. Current research is looking at better ways to fix the artificial hip and to prevent wear of the components, which can ultimately lead to failure, especially for hip replacements performed at an early age.

Although hip replacement is almost thought of as routine in an orthopaedic surgical hospital, it is nevertheless a major operation and one not to be undertaken lightly. For this reason Dr Trahair's book plays a vital role in explaining what is it actually like to undergo joint replacement surgery from a patient perspective. Many booklets have been published in this field, but they have mainly been written by surgeons for patients, not by patients for other patients. Dr Trahair takes the reader in chronological order through the journey from first symptoms to the post-operative follow-up many months after the surgery. Along the way he gives an accurate account of both his own and other patients' feelings about how they approached the decision to have a hip replacement, their time in hospital, and recuperating after the operation. There are many personal accounts of patients' own feelings, and I, as a hip surgeon, found them particularly informative. The helpful glossary explains some of the terms frequently used in association with joint replacement.

I am sure readers will find this a well-written and very informative guide to hip replacement. I thoroughly recommend this book to those people contemplating a new hip.

Richard de Steiger
MB, BS, FRACS (Orth.)
Orthopaedic surgeon

Contents

Acknowledgments

I am indebted to many friends and colleagues who helped me to find people who were willing to talk about their lives before, during, and after the hip operation. I am also grateful to friends who are experts in the various branches of medicine and were willing to pass on impressions of how they manage patients as they go about their work.

For this book transcripts of interviews were typed by Heather Eather, and help in finding informants who were unknown to me came from Katy Richmond, Lyn Baker, Carol Dobbin, Russ Newton, Gill Tucker, and Libby Tronson. The reference staff at the Borchardt Library, La Trobe University, provided excellent service in searching for relevant sources on hip replacement. The book benefited greatly from the help of Sue Berry, David Bracy, Paula Darling, Janine Dobyn, Wendy Edde, Cathryn Game, Richard Harper, Geoffrey Littlejohn, Champak Rana, Peter Rose, Marion Severn, Mitchell Smith, Richard de Steiger, and Richard Travers.

I am most grateful to my thirteen informants, all of whom had new hips. For each informant I have chosen a pseudonym as we agreed. A biography of each informant is provided at the back of the book.

All words in **bold type** are explained in the glossary.

Introduction

This book is for people who are thinking about having a new hip. Based on the experiences of fourteen patients, the book tells of life before the operation, the decision to have a new hip, preparation for life in hospital, and recovery afterwards. With the patients' experiences, the book integrates the expectations and advice on hip replacement from surgeons, rheumatologists, physiotherapists, nurses, and occupational therapists.

A medical acquaintance once said to me that most people who are about to have a new hip ask only two questions: What will it cost? How long will I be out of action?

For Australian patients who are not insured, the operation costs between $20,000 and $40,000, depending on your surgeon. In Australia, if you are fully insured you should expect to pay between $600 and $1200. In Great Britain and Australia the cost is about half that in the USA; in Hong Kong it is almost twice that of the USA.

You will be out of action for between eight and ten weeks. Of that period two weeks will be spent in hospital, and four to six weeks will be spent recovering at home. You can expect another two to pass before you will be able to drive yourself. So allow at least eight weeks away from work.

If you are fully insured you will probably have to spend about five weeks preparing yourself for the operation in a private hospital. If you are not fully insured you will probably have to have an operation in a public hospital, where, according to one doctor, there will be a waiting period of between six months and two years because the operation is not regarded as essential.

In the mid 1990s world wide more than half a million new hips were given to people who suffered from arthritis and related diseases; of these about 130,000 were in the USA and about 20,000 in Australia. Since the mid 1980s the success rate of new hips has risen greatly — well over 90 per cent — and most people who have a new hip can look forward to at least ten years without pain. The success rate is not so high among people who need to have their new hip replaced, but even that operation is enjoying an improved rate of success today.

The main reason for having a new hip is to rid yourself of severe pain and to increase your ability to get about in comfort. Without a new hip most sufferers would finish in a wheelchair as they did before World War II. There are other ways to manage pain in the hip, but most simply delay the inevitable operation.

The operation is serious, a 'brute of a thing', as one of my informants said. It takes about ninety minutes. You are completely out to it for a short period beforehand and for many hours afterwards. The shock to the body is great, and most patients are naturally frightened by the thought of the operation. The alternative — continued pain, increased use of painkiller, and life in a wheelchair — makes the decision very clear, if not easy.

Recuperation from the operation is frustrating because full recovery can take many months — even a year or so — but the result is rewarding for most sufferers because the pain evaporates, life becomes worth living, and your friends and relatives see you happy again.

The length of the recovery depends very much on you, how well you prepared for the operation, life in hospital, and the health gains made later. Two kinds of preparation are helpful: (1) improving your health before the operation and planning for your home life during your the recovery; and (2) reducing the natural fear and anxiety about the operation itself. If you are well prepared both physically and in yourself, your recovery will be rapid and effortless.

This book blends the experiences of patients with the expectations of medical experts. It is no substitute for medical advice. Among my informants only one was a doctor. The remainder were like me, uncertain, uninformed, and anxious about getting a new hip. They included nurses, a politician, several teachers, an architect, a restaurant owner, an art gallery director, a bus driver, and two students. They gave their time, much careful thought, and frank replies to my questions. I was grateful and pleased to hear what they had to say, to compare their experiences with my own, and to enjoy the articulate way in which they told me their stories.

In this book the account of what medical experts expect of you as a patient comes from the sources listed in the selected reading.

The first chapter tells how I and each of my informants came to suffer from pain in the hip, how we diagnosed our complaints, and finally had to accept the fact that we had arthritis in one of its many forms. This is followed by a short account of what arthritis appears to be, its uncertain origins, and some methods of managing it. The second chapter summarises the course taken by my informants to find a surgeon and to decide if and when to have a new hip. Chapter 3 describes how the informants learned to become patients for a hip operation and considers the cost of the operation, making plans to go to hospital, choosing a hospital, preparing your health for the operation, deciding whose blood to use, managing pain before the operation, preparing your home for the recovery, useful aids for comfortable recovering, the pre-admission clinic, and anxiety about being a patient.

Chapter 4 outlines what you can expect to happen when you get to the hospital and settle in for the operation, meet the people who will be helping you, learn what happens and wake up after the operation. The first two or three days after the operation from the patients' viewpoint, and what the hospital staff anticipate generally, are described in chapter 5. Attention centres on how you sleep, your pain and how it gradually goes, and how your body begins to function as it did before the operation. In chapter 6 hospital life takes on a different meaning as you recover, get out of bed and walk again. The recovery begins to take a clear path, although there are some minor problems for some people on the way. In chapter 7 life begins at home again as you learn how to recover faster and to manage several weeks of slowly becoming less dependent on others. Many precautions are taken, and much thought is given to recovering securely. The next chapter describes problems and complications that affect the rate of recovery and what you can expect in the years after the operation. The last chapter summarises decisions that patients made and actions they took to become free of pain and begin life with a new hip.

'My hip's a bit of a worry'

Personal histories of hip trouble

Early in 1992 I had a persistent pain near the outer edge of my left hip. Thinking it was a pain in my lower back that had flared up once more, I did my usual exercises, but it did not go away. I decided to forget the discomfort. By November 1992 I could no longer ignore the pain. I went to the medical officer at the university where I work and was X-rayed. The medical officer showed me that the gap between my left thigh bone — my **femur** — and the hip bone — my **acetabulum** — was becoming narrow, and the gap was surrounded by inflammation. (Words in **bold type** are explained in the glossary.) He said the inflammation was **arthritis**. This was grim news to me. He showed me that inflammation was also growing around the right hip joint. Perhaps in a few years much the same discomfort would occur there too. Things were getting worse. What could I do?

I felt responsible for the arthritis, and I had to find the right treatment. I took up swimming and a tablet of a prescribed **anti-inflammatory drug** each day. I did not swim regularly. Tablets worked very well. I felt that my arthritis had gone. In case it had not, I continued taking the tablets because I did not have time to be concerned about whether the pain would return. I kept up the exercises to strengthen my stomach muscles and lower back, and felt I was back in control of my health.

A year later I was working in a small beach-side town in the USA. One night after watching TV, I rose quickly from the couch. Suddenly a muscle spasm clutched the inside of my left leg. I diagnosed the problem immediately — severe cramp — and applied the usual remedies. Might it be something else? Something serious? In three minutes all was well, the cramp had gone, and — again being an expert in medical diagnosis — I decided the pain was due simply to the fact that I had not been exercising as often as I should have been. So at four o'clock each day I would stop writing and walk through the town and along the beach.

The pain in the hip became worse. I could not stand easily. After a few days without the tablets, I ached in other places. For relief at the end of the day I took another whisky. I did not like the pain and increasing the use of whisky so liberally. It is depressing to be in pain and need tablets and alcohol. Maybe I should walk more? Walking was a good exercise, but it took about ten minutes walking before the pain eased, and the pain came back when I stood up.

In the Australian summer of 1995 I had had enough. A fresh set of X-rays and a **CT scan** of my back showed that I would need a new left hip. Should I have a new hip now? My general practitioner suggested that I see a specialist about my lower back first because the pain in my left side might be due to a disc pressing on the **sciatic nerve**. Then perhaps I should try a **physiotherapist**.

The **orthopaedic surgeon** scanned the image of my precious spine on the screen, ordered me to lie on his couch, and tested my reflexes in the ankles and knees. He advised: 'Best thing to do is to see the physio, play golf, and if you have any difficulty with your back then we can operate to relieve the pain there.' Wonderful news!

At the physiotherapist's rooms I lay on a narrow table while he began to massage the inner left thigh, to stretch the muscles, and to open the hip so that my leg rolled outwards away from my body. He showed me various stretching exercises, which I felt were impossible. He said they would become easier as I tried them each day at home, and that I should walk briskly for fifteen minutes, night and morning.

In a few days I found myself a little more nimble than in the past. After ten weeks of massaging and stretching I joined a weekly early morning group to do the exercises with people who were in similar trouble. I felt so much better. I was sure I had conquered the hip problem. I began going to two early morning groups each week. The results were so gratifying that I swore I would make them part of my everyday life from that day forward.

But when I went on vacation in summer and neglected the stretching, the pain returned, and the tablets were not working as they had been. I knew I was still in a bad way.

A doctor friend recommended a **rheumatologist**, who agreed that a hip replacement was imminent, but advised me to wait as long as I could because people who were younger than 60 were a little too young. Hip replacement, he said, might last about fifteen years. Put the operation off so that you do not have to have it done again, was his advice. I agreed, but in a few months I had had enough of the pain and decided to see a surgeon.

The experience of others

Bernard

Bernard, 64, drives a school bus in the country. Like his brother, he found he was becoming immobilised because of his hip and in much pain with arthritis.

> "The doctor prescribed anti-inflammatory tablets and showed me the X-rays. My leg bone was a bit flat on the top. In a month the bones had gone from being a sixteenth of an inch apart to bone mashed on bone. I couldn't put on my socks without a struggle."

Betty

Betty, a retired school teacher in her mid eighties, was born with one leg shorter than the other, and for many years had an **orthotic** in her shoe. She had no pain until she was in her sixties.

> "I noticed that I had pain in the base of the spine. I was leaning over a bathroom sink when my back locked. In the seventies not very much was done about hips. Since then I've had pain. The trouble began with my back, never my hip, until the nineties."

Betty had no problem about accepting the need for a new hip, but she was not happy with the surgeon her doctor had recommended.

"I just felt I wouldn't want him cutting into me, and I said, 'I don't want to go back to him, please.' I thought he was a bit supercilious. He made me reveal myself, and he commented more on my knee. And he said, 'I think you'd just better wait and see how you go for the rest of the year. Come to me if you think you need the operation.' Well, I'd damn well gone to him because I needed an operation! I didn't stop to argue with him. You have to have confidence in your doctor. My doctor said, 'I've got a good man, but further away.' He was quite right."

Charles

Charles, 64, is a former politician. He writes occasionally for newspapers and pursues scholarly interests. All his life he had exercised and looked after his health. Some years ago he pulled a muscle rather severely while waterskiing.

"I felt some restriction in movement in the right leg when I chased the ball on the tennis court, but I didn't relate it to any problem of the hip. I used to notice some pain after exercise, after playing tennis. I used to jog four or five mornings a week for thirty-five years. Thumped around a squash court for about fifteen years in my twenties, thirties, and forties. So I put in a lot of groundwork to wreck the hip. It was the fashion for our generation. If you hadn't done all that exercise you might well have had a heart attack at 35."

About two years ago he went to see a physiotherapist about a lower back complaint. He could not raise his leg easily. X-rays showed that his hip was in trouble, and it deteriorated quickly. He stopped running and tennis, and turned to cycling and swimming. Within twelve months he was struggling to get up stairs. He saw a surgeon who encouraged him to wait until the pain was more severe. Charles held himself responsible for his hip trouble.

"It was my lack of circumspection about exercise. So I think I've done it myself. So far as I am aware, neither my mother nor my father had any problems, and they both lived full lives. I have an older sister; she didn't have trouble."

In pain and worried, Charles knew that a hip replacement was imminent. He allayed his anxiety by investigating it as best he could. Meanwhile he used mild treatment.

"I took those anti-inflammatories for a while. They're not terribly good for some people's stomachs. I used them very sparingly, and in the end I just didn't use them at all because the side effects were not worth it. In the end I got tired of it. I found a way I could sleep. And I knew what I could do and what I couldn't do. Of course, what happens when you become aware that you're going to have an operation is that you hear the stories about the operations. The range of things you hear about makes your imagination start to work. It becomes important to be reassured. I investigated hip replacements. A very good friend in a medical family helped by recommending that I see somebody else. I was very confident that he would point me in the right direction. And once I'd talked to a couple of specialists about it I felt quite good."

Doug

Doug, 53, a university architect, had slight cerebral palsy down his right leg. When he was 50 he had a persistent pain in his knee and noticed muscle wastage in his leg although he was a vigorous cyclist.

"Having all this exercise — 26 kilometres a day on the bike — how can I still get muscle wastage and problems with the knee? Must be something to do with the cerebral palsy."

He saw a specialist whose advice seemed irrelevant. Three years later — after following a philosophy of 'no pain no gain', and playing two rounds of golf a day rather than one, and in increasing pain from walking — Doug had his knee X-rayed.

"I found that the pain wasn't being transmitted from the knee, where there was slight arthritis, but from the hip. There was just bone on bone and no **cartilage** between the bones. It was very surprising to me to find out that it was my hip. Apparently it was not caused by the cerebral palsy as such but by the fact that the cerebral palsy had made me flat-footed on one side, and I was a centimetre shorter in the right leg. All the walking and jogging, which I thought was doing me good, was actually compounding the problem. The difference in the legs had a jarring and hammering effect on the separation in the hip between the ball and the socket. Finally it was bone on bone, with more restriction in movement, and more pain."

Doug saw a specialist, who confirmed the diagnosis that his hip needed replacement. Doug was surprised that the surgeon recommended the operation for one so young.

"I was only 52. I had just started back at work on the building site at the university, and I was under very big pressure, so I couldn't see myself having six weeks off. So I asked if would I be doing any harm to myself by continuing for some time. He said I wouldn't be, and that eventually pain would bring me back because the hip joint had gone anyway."

At a local science museum Doug saw different types of hip **prosthesis**.

"Because I am at a university, I have access to the biomedical library, which carries videotapes of nearly every operation that's undertaken. I could have got a videotape and watched a hip operation. I didn't want to do that. Didn't want to make myself more apprehensive."

Ernst

Ernst, 45, a psychiatrist and an accomplished hammer thrower, had gained a place in the Olympic training team in 1980. Recently he had two operations, one on each hip, with only three months between them. He first became aware of his hip trouble ten years earlier when pain affected his running. He had a slight congenital malformation of the hips such that the socket of the hip, **acetabula fossa**, was too shallow for the head of the femur. Consequently the latter hung out a little. For twenty-five years he had not crossed his legs; he was unable to stand easily with his feet together or do up his shoes. He dreaded going to a cocktail party, because he could cope for only twenty minutes and then had to find a seat.

Ernst had known he was a candidate for two new hips and brought his medical expertise to the problem.

"I read extensively. I am a bit obsessive about things. I went through medical school with my surgeon, a personal friend, and I just phoned him. I'd assisted in hip replacements when I was a junior doctor. I also went through medical journals and got articles on hips. I also got a book that confirmed a lot of stuff I already knew."

Fred

Fred, 70, is a retired academic and had a hip operation two years ago. Twenty years earlier he was in England, and he went to see his general practitioner because of persistent pain in his right hip. X-rays showed that Fred's hip was so arthritic that bone was grinding on bone. To relieve the pain the general practitioner prescribed an anti-inflammatory drug. Before taking the drug Fred investigated it, and decided he preferred the pain to a drug with such deleterious side effects. Twenty years later, in great pain and using a stick to steady himself, Fred decided enough was enough. His general practitioner in Australia recommended that he see two surgeons and decide on an operation to get a new hip.

Helen

Helen, a New Zealander in her mid twenties, has had six hip operations, and today she is not certain what they all were for. The pain started in 1980, and she was about 11 when the first operation was done. She had a series of operations during her teenage years.

She had started to have hip pains when walking in Papua New Guinea where she was with her mother, an anthropologist. In Papua New Guinea she was diagnosed as having bone cancer, so the family rushed her back to New Zealand for further examinations. They discovered she did not have bone cancer, but the doctors didn't know what her illness was. Soon she was bent double. She was sent to hospital, put in traction for eight weeks, and given drugs. To straighten her back she was put in a cast from her upper body down one side of one leg. Later she was put in a brace, and finally she was given tranquillisers and diagnosed as suffering from some psychosomatic disorder. Her mother disagreed. The family returned to Papua New Guinea for six months and then decided to go to Australia, where Helen was diagnosed as having **rheumatoid arthritis**.

"The arthritis had progressed a lot and occurred in both hips. There was not much left of them. Doctors were uncertain about doing an operation on someone so young. I was written up in the Mayo Clinic journal for being the youngest hip replacement at that time so it was fairly ground-breaking. And it was done mainly because Mum did an enormous amount of research into hip replacements. All the **synovial fluid** between the hip joint and the femur had completely disappeared, and the bones had rubbed each other down so that there was no hope of repair. First, they wanted to pin the hip, and I wouldn't have been able to bend properly, because I would have been straight along one side. But my mother read all the medical journals, talked to doctors, and was ready to counter their arguments with the latest procedures just to save my capacity to walk."

Mario

Mario, 57, and his wife operate a small restaurant in the country. Five years ago he had a new left hip and now he feels the other hip needs similar attention. He has **haemochromatosis**, that is, too much iron in his blood, which gives him a propensity to arthritis. For relief he also takes a prescribed anti-inflammatory drug.

> "The pain began in the knees and in the ankles, and it seemed to start with the joints before it became muscular. I was exploring all sorts of possibilities. I didn't think that it could've been my hip. I went to various people, and I didn't get any lasting relief. They ranged from Chinese herbalists to some more way-out manipulators. Ultimately the pain became localised in the hip, and it was very difficult to walk. It was difficult to stand after I'd been sitting for a while. It wasn't a continuous pain — it came and went."

Mario is worried that he might need to have an operation on the right hip as well.

> "At the present I'm noticing more pain in the back than the hip, and in the back of the thigh bone, up high, and not so much from the actual **pelvis**. Having had the hip operation, I knew virtually from the first pains that it was coming through again. I went to a specialist, and X-rays were taken. The evidence was there. Because of the pain the most sensible thing to do seemed to be to get it treated. I didn't like what I imagined it would be. If you don't get a new hip you suffer a lot of pain and you lack mobility. I did all the diagnosis, and planned how to recover. I thought, 'No, there's nothing the matter with my hip.' You go through that. That's very natural. You don't want to accept the trouble in your hip. The pain comes and goes, and because these things give you some relief, you think, 'Ah, that's all it was.' "

Nell

Nell, in her fifties, had had arthritis for many years in her neck, shoulders, and spine. She used various anti-inflammatories for relief, and remarked that she and her dog used the same drug for arthritis pain. She had the operation very soon after her pain became severe.

> "The pain seemed to come on very quickly. About a year before that I actually felt odd pains in the right hip when I was walking. I had arranged

to go overseas with friends, and I went. I was very determined to go. It wasn't awfully clever of me because my walking deteriorated so much so quickly that I had to get a stick."

At first, she was sent to a surgeon she did not warm to.

"He grabbed my leg and twisted it upside down and round about. He caused quite a bit of pain, so much so that I felt it for two days afterwards. There's no way I'm going back to him. He had a good name, but when I complained to my doctor, she said, 'Well, he can be a bit rough.' An old friend, a physiotherapist, suggested another specialist because she'd worked with him before. I couldn't speak highly enough of him. He was marvellous. I didn't have physiotherapy. I did see a doctor at one stage, and he said, 'You'd better do some exercise and build up the muscles because you're going to need them afterwards.' "

Sonomi

Sonomi, 57, a busy art gallery director, originally from the USA, developed lower back pain about ten years go. She tried exercises and physiotherapy. After about six years her general practitioner suggested seeing a rheumatologist, who said she would need a new hip. Sonomi had a problem choosing a surgeon. She saw more than one. Finally she chose the surgeon whom she thought had the most considerate manner. She waited a little more than three years before having the operation and recently came home to recover.

Terri

Terri is in her mid thirties. At 14 she learned she had rheumatoid arthritis. She used to ride horses, and found she couldn't extend her leg sideways.

"When I was riding, I felt a muscle was in need of stretching, and that was obviously the start of it. I actually had signs of it even earlier than that, but I didn't know, and my doctor didn't know. The middle joint on my index finger swelled up, and my doctor thought I had sprained it. Then my wrist joint become swollen and later went away. Twelve months later everything started hurting. The onset of pain was really quick — within about six weeks."

Drugs were used to treat her swellings. She went to hospital and was put to bed, wearing splints all day, for six weeks.

"Since then I've been on drug therapy. I've had the arthritis for almost twenty years now. I have **osteoporosis** as well, which often happens after you've had rheumatoid arthritis for any length of time, and I've also suffered with **endometriosis**."

Terri was unprepared for the shock of a hip operation.

"In my mid twenties my rheumatologist said, 'Well, you've got arthritis in the hips, you've got secondary osteoporosis. One day you're going to have to have a hip replacement.' I just burst into tears. It was the first time I'd ever cried in front of my rheumatologist, and I'd been seeing him since I was 14. I remember his words vividly. 'Don't worry. When the time comes to have the operation, you'll be ready for it emotionally because you'll be desperate to have it.' It was very true."

Meanwhile, Terri found an unusual way to manage the pain.

"I was involved in a church in my late twenties and for spiritual reasons I did a lengthy fast of forty days. I had to take some milk with my medication, but apart from that I was on a water fast. I had great success with that. It almost arrested the symptoms. I did it also to detoxify my body. After that fast I did things like rock climbing that I'd never done before. I almost had no pain. I came off the pain-relief drugs, but I stayed on the long-term anti-inflammatories. It was such an achievement."

Tess

Tess, 85, had three operations on the same hip. In her youth she had been a theatre nurse, and attributed her hip problems to that work.

"I didn't have any trouble inside the hip at all when I was standing and walking and lifting it into the car. I hadn't fractured it, I hadn't fallen. I think it was because of the way I stood up. I used to stand all day in the operating theatre. It became impacted because of that. The surgeon didn't say it was a badly arthritic hip at all, but it was impacted. Something I brought on myself."

She went to the doctor happy to be getting rid of the discomfort, not thinking her hip needed replacement. She waited two years before her surgeon wanted to operate. By then she was 70. When she was 78 the pain returned in her thigh.

"When I went to turn over in bed I could feel that one part of my leg went, and the other didn't. There was a sort of grinding sound. I went into my surgeon, and he said the cement used to secure the prosthesis had cracked."

How did the cement crack? She recalled two events that she thought might have been responsible.

"When we were on holidays in England, my heel caught in the metal strip in somebody's doorway, and I sort of flew across the hall. Bumped myself badly. I didn't feel any ill-effect at the time. Another time when we were on holidays, I popped in quickly to change my shoes, sat on the bed — which had a slippery counterpane — and slipped straight on to the floor. BANG! When I got up I felt I hadn't actually fallen on the hip. Again, the accident didn't have any ill-effects at the time. Either fall could've cracked it."

Suddenly, about twelve months later, she knew something was wrong. Complications followed the second operation, and a third, which left her with a limp, was needed. Tess relied on the reputation of the hospital and the surgeon.

"The hospital he used was the place to go in those days. The third floor had a very good name for orthopaedic surgery. My surgeon was one of the best ones. My own doctor sent me to him. Didn't go to others. Didn't shop around or read any medical journals."

Wendy

Wendy, 52, a mother and housewife, had once been a nurse. On the day her hero, Betty Cuthbert, was running in the 1956 Melbourne Olympics, Wendy was 12. She ran to her aunt's house after school to watch Betty race because her family didn't have TV.

"Well, I didn't make it. I was run over by a council truck. My pelvis and my right leg were crushed. So the head of my right femur didn't develop in a smooth way like the left one. It was rough, and it wasn't getting an adequate supply of blood. It had much the same effect as an arthritic hip."

At the age of 21 Wendy had much discomfort in her right hip.

"At the time in England they were only starting to do modern hip replacements. I was advised to wait for techniques to improve, and to hold out as long as I could."

She went to England to further her nursing skills and was warned not to get a new hip, so she didn't. She married and had five children; the last two were twins. All her pregnancies strained her right hip.

"There was pain, but I suppose because you're pretty resilient as a child, and you want to do the same things as everyone else, I did build up a pretty good pain tolerance. I was always aware that I had to make myself last as long as possible."

Trouble in the hip

The stories of hip trouble centre on the emergence of pain so great that the sufferer cannot get adequate relief and a doctor's advice is needed. The pain seems to emerge from the leg, the hip and/or the back, but eventually is traced to the hip. Why is that?

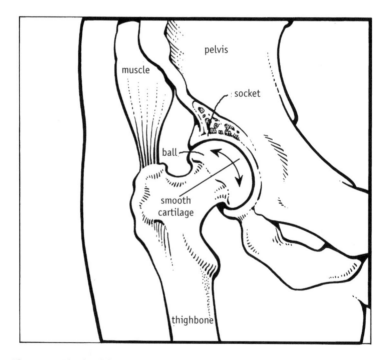

Figure 1: The healthy hip. The ball and socket fit closely, the cartilage is smooth, and the hip is held in place by muscles and ligaments.

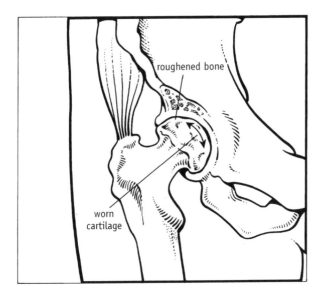

Figure 2: A problem hip. The cartilage is worn, the head of the femur is rough, the muscle is in spasm, and movement is painful and restricted.

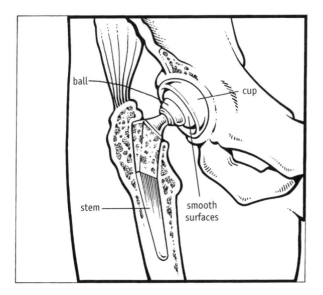

Figure 3: Hip replacement. The head of the femur is a titanium ball, the socket of the acetabulum is tough, smooth plastic, and the new hip is held by a stem fitted down the thigh bone.

The hip is a set of bones or a joint that links our spine with our legs. It does so through a ball-and-socket system. The ball is at the top of the thigh bone, or femur; the socket is on the outer side of the pelvic bone, or acetabulum. Inside the acetabulum is a cartilage layer; another is on the head of the femur. The ball and the socket fit closely, and are lubricated by a grease-like fluid, synovial fluid, protected by a strong layer of gristle, and held in place by ligaments, a tough membrane, and our muscles. By the time we are adolescents this ball-and-socket joint has developed fully. The hip operates with a rich supply of blood and a powerful network of nerves.

Normally the ball and socket can be bent (called **flexion**), straightened (**extension**), and twisted or rotated externally or internally, lifted sideways so our legs are apart (**abduction**). We can also cross our legs (**adduction**).

When the hip is in trouble, or diseased, these normal movements are severely curtailed, sometimes impossible. How does that happen? The strong muscles all around the hip go into spasm and in time shorten (called **contracture**). For most of us with trouble in the hip the main problem is **flexion contracture**. So we find the hip joint becomes less and less flexible, might take ages to straighten when we stand up, and hurt when we play a sport, ride a horse, jog, walk up stairs, or swing a golf club. This is what happened to me, Betty, Doug, Fred, Mario, Sonomi, and Terri. Not in the same way, or for the same reason — but the intense pain emerged for us all.

We suffered from a disease of the hip, arthritis, which placed a painful stress on our hip. The movement of our hip was so greatly curtailed that discomfort and pain emerged not only in the hip's ball and socket but also in the knees and the lower back. We had great difficulty deciding what was the matter, frequently concluded that our knees, thighs, and back were in trouble, and, with this false self-diagnosis, went ahead and exercised in a way that made the hip worse.

Arthritis

What is arthritis, and what is pain doing to us? The pain is a natural way of alerting us to the fact that we need to do something about the trouble in the hip. Arthritis is what leads us to suffer the trouble in the hip. Arthritis comes in many forms, but the two most common are **osteoarthritis** and rheumatoid arthritis. Another common group comprises **spondylitis,** and **gout**, and there are rarities such as multiple **epiphysial dysplasia**, in which not all joints develop. Among the many varieties the first two emerged clearly with my informants. Rheumatoid arthritis plagued the lives of Helen and Terri, while osteoarthritis affected the other people.

Why do we get arthritis? Each sufferer had a guess. Wendy's arthritis arose because of an accident with the council truck and the subsequent malformation of her hip; Ernst had a congenital hip problem, which was heritable; Betty and Doug had similar causes; Charles seemed to have bludgeoned his hip with over-exercise, while Tess's work might have contributed to her suffering originally. Tracing the origins of arthritis is as difficult as deciding how many forms it takes.

Arthritis is inflammation of joints. They become inflamed due largely to wear and tear. Arthritis emerges among older people, those who are much overweight, and some who have suffered some injury, like Wendy. This is osteoarthritis. Rheumatoid arthritis affects many parts of the body, mainly the joints, but is found in the heart, kidneys, and tendons as well. Inflammation, the cause of pain, occurs at the joints, subjecting the sufferer to dreadful stiffness and to swellings that come and go. Usually rheumatoid arthritis affects young women.

Osteoarthritis

Osteoarthritis is common among all animals and has been for all time. Early human hip bones show evidence of the disease. Today this disease increases in incidence with age. More than half of us who are 40 or older have some experience of it in the weight-bearing joints where our cartilage begins to flake.

Two groups of osteoarthritis have been identified. **Primary osteoarthritis**, whose origins are not securely known, is thought by some doctors to start in the smaller joints like the hands and progress to other larger joints, such as the knees and hips. In the experience of other doctors there is no such progress, and they report primary osteoarthritis in both small and large joints independently. Sometimes primary osteoarthritis appears quickly, and it is often found in women after menopause. **Secondary osteo-arthritis** is due to an old injury, a birth defect, or some infection or disease in the hip. Such arthritis might be due also to diseases of the nervous system like syphilis; areas where the bone dies due to lack of blood (**avascular necrosis**), anti-inflammatory drugs, alcoholism, or getting the bends; metabolic disorders, like gout; and rare nutritional disorders.

Rheumatoid arthritis

Helen and Terri suffered from rheumatoid arthritis. Helen had it in the distressing juvenile form. In these cases many joints are affected by inflammation of the **synovium**; pain appears in the morning and towards the end of the day. Sufferers feel very tired and ill. Their arthritis involves unusually fragile bones that erode easily. This makes hip operations hazardous, but often in these cases an operation is all that can be offered.

Coping with arthritis

How do you cope with arthritis? From the sufferer's point of view, the trouble in the hip is accompanied by **chronic pain**, that is, pain that lasts more than two to three months and calls for some physical treatment. We curb our activities to relieve the pain. Thus our lifestyle changes. We stiffen up, cannot play or work as we once did, and generally we do not enjoy things as much as we used to.

Why do we have such chronic pain? Chronic pain generally arises from stress, and is accompanied by variations in blood pressure, palpitations (real or imagined), and stomach trouble. Such complaints as these tend to make us even more unhappy and worried, and can lead us into highly irritable, sad, and even depressed states. What do we do? We take or do something for the trouble. We try to get rid of it with **analgesic** painkillers, sedatives to put us at ease, muscle relaxants like alcohol, prescribed anti-inflammatory drugs, and even **narcotics**.

But drugs have side effects such as drowsiness, dizziness, blurred vision, stomach upsets, liver damage, **insomnia**, and occasional swellings, and often our depression deepens. As we use different drugs to counter this side effect of pain treatment, often we have more stomach complaints; we might find the heart, lungs, and general circulation are affected; blood pressure mounts or falls; sexual and other libidinal interests are impaired; and we go into a decline and become different characters. And people say to us 'You are not yourself today.' And we feel even worse because we feel that our attempts have failed to make us feel better.

We try other ways. We dash off to some fashionable experts, decide it is diet, not exercise, that is the trouble, or vice versa, try another form of medicine from another culture, give up exercise for meditation, jogging for deep breathing, yoga for eating a high-protein diet, and so on. Such attempts at self-diagnosis and treatment usually fail. And for this reason, at some stage, we turn to professional medical advice.

First, from medical advice we learn that pain arises from many causes and that it might be related to chemical inadequacies in what we eat. Maybe you will learn that the cause of pain might be deficiencies — vitamins A to E, calcium, magnesium, or zinc. Such insufficiency might check the supply of synovial fluid to the joints, and thus prevent their adequate lubrication and cause our stiffness and pain. Such dietary deficiencies could be why our muscles go into spasm, and why we get pains in the neck, shoulder, back, hip, and even **angina** of the heart. Perhaps the distress we feel is made worse by a lack of vitamin C; maybe B-complex vitamins are needed to make our nervous system healthier, because inadequate supplies can lead to heart disease, irritability, and depression.

Third, from doctors and paramedical experts we also learn that other treatments can help with chronic arthritis. They can advise you on the use of exercises with physiotherapists that release natural opiate-like substances, that is, **endorphins** related to pain suppression. Some people respond favourably to **hypnosis**, and to learning self-hypnosis and other meditative techniques of pain control. Others learn to alter their diet to use only fresh foods and cease using bacon, beer, caffeinated drinks, processed meat, canned or otherwise, marinated and pickled foods, MSG, canned soups and frozen dinners, salami, smoked fish and meat, wine and champagne, yeast and yeast extracts. Other well-recommended mild forms of treatment are **homoeopathy**, **osteopathy**, and **acupuncture**.

Mild forms of treatment sometimes achieve considerable success. In my case stretching, combined with the use of a prescribed anti-inflammatory drug, produced great relief. The drug had no effects on my stomach — although it did affect friends who used it briefly — and stretching under supervision of a physiotherapist eased the pain considerably.

I found these two treatments were techniques of delay and comfort. Stretching and anti-inflammatories were mild forms of managing the pain, and they had limits as the wear on my hip progressed. A radical form of treatment was called for. The deep pain of bone grinding on bone was too much, or, as my rheumatologist muttered, 'It's a lifestyle problem for you.'

(2)

Choosing the surgeon and making the decision

How should you decide on a surgeon? A medical friend gave me a name and an address, and even recommended a hospital. I had not heard of the surgeon or the hospital, but when I mentioned them to other friends they nodded in approval. I then returned to the rheumatologist and advised him that I wanted to see a surgeon. He hesitated. I said my mind was made up. I did not want the pain any more. I made it clear to him that in so many ways it was interfering with my life.

The anti-inflammatory tablets were having little effect. I could sit quite comfortably, but when I stood to cross the room it was almost a minute before the left leg would reach to the floor. I limped badly, and attracted all kinds of advice and occasionally embarrassing sympathy. Young people suggested swimming; old people said go to bed. The rheumatologist agreed that since I was at the age of 60 I was ready. Before he could come up with the name of a surgeon I quickly gave him the name of the man who had been recommended to me. He immediately agreed. So that was it. The surgeon could see me in three weeks.

I gave him the story I have so far told. In a business-like and brusque manner he told me to walk along the hallway. When I returned he said that I was in enough trouble to be a candidate for a new hip. In the X-rays he showed that the pain was caused largely by the flattening of the head of the femur and the grinding of bone on bone in my hip socket. He seemed to think that the right side was not as serious as the left, and that there might not be any need to operate on the right hip.

I made the decision then. I felt there was no alternative but to have the operation. I did not want my hip to get any worse, and I knew that there was nothing more I could do to ease the pain. The stretching exercises had been most beneficial; the tablets did help but only a little. My hip could only become worse. I wanted to walk normally again, to play golf, and move about easily. Unless I had the operation I would not be able to do any of these things.

The surgeon said the benefit would be increased flexibility and mobility and less pain. He recommended that my own blood be used for the operation. I had no wish to learn about the details of the operation, or the **anaesthetic**, and did not ask him for any information about what would happen to me.

What would be the disadvantages of having an operation? My surgeon said there were three: first, I could get an **infection**; second, the hip could become dislocated; third, I could get a **blood clot** in the leg, which could threaten my life. These threats were serious, so special precautions were normally taken. To prevent infection the operating theatre was thoroughly sterilised, and every effort was made to prevent infection occurring in the wound. Of course nothing was 100 per cent guaranteed. I understood that. To prevent **dislocation** I would be kept on a special regimen after the operation. He gave no details. Finally, to prevent blood from clotting, various measures would be followed and special tablets taken, and I would be under close supervision. I did not think to ask if there were any other dangers or disadvantages to having an operation, and he did not volunteer any further information about the dangers of being a patient having a total hip replacement. But, as he pointed to the X-ray on the wall beside his desk, he did say that my bones were healthy and strong. That comment was reassuring, and I felt that recovery would not be a problem.

I wanted to know how long I would be out of action. I had planned to be abroad in ten weeks time to speak at a conference. He assured me that I could be there. The operation would require me to be in hospital for ten to fourteen days. Then I would convalesce for four weeks. Thereafter I would be able to get about and drive a car again. It seemed I would be out of normal operation for about six to eight weeks.

The surgeon took me to his nurse–secretary, saying that she would tell me about the costs, and left her to make the appointments. Just as he turned to go, he gave me a friendly poke me in the stomach and said cheerily: 'Better lose a bit of that.' His nurse, in an equally cheery way, disagreed. But by the time she had spoken he was out of earshot.

The plans were made. The nurse and I set the date for the operation at the private hospital my medical friend had mentioned. I had about a month to wait.

Bernard

As his hip became more painful Bernard began to think he would soon be in a wheelchair and not be able to drive the school bus. The surgeon asked Bernard to consider the question of having an operation carefully.

> "The surgeon said, 'You want to think about this. Things could happen. Infection can set in, and there are no guarantees, you know.' I suppose they've got to tell you these things. The other thing that could happen was blood clotting."

He had been given a choice of surgeons by his general practitioner and made the choice after talking with his daughter. His brother recommended against the operation and suggested exercises instead.

> "My brother said, 'Don't have it done.' I think he did the wrong thing. He went and drove tractors too soon after the operation and I don't think his hip is quite right."

The pain was too much for Bernard to accept his brother's advice.

> "The day I went to see the surgeon the wife came in with me, and, of course, I had to strip off, and she virtually had to take my socks off for me."

The surgeon showed Bernard the prosthesis that would be put into his femur and acetabulum.

"It was just like a stainless steel ball they have in the steering of the car. He said that in the early days in some of the operations, the steel wasn't as good as it is today. He showed me one that had a crack right through it. It was a piece of steel as thick as your finger."

Bernard also discussed the outcome of the operation with others, and they encouraged him to have it.

"They said, 'Oh, so-and-so had that, and it's marvellous, you know.' I went to the local private hospital and had it in the middle of October."

Betty

Betty saw a specialist who said he did not know whether her problem lay in the back or the hip. To reach her apartment, she told him, she had to mount thirty-two steps, and the climb was becoming increasingly difficult. He advised waiting twelve months. Before the time was up she found the pain unbearable. It came from anywhere between her hip and her knee. A second specialist she saw ten months later said he had no choice but to replace her hip.

"He didn't give me any advice. He said he couldn't take me for three months, then he flew off overseas. He didn't have much to do with me at all. He didn't tell me about any risks. I think they usually take them and do the best they can. I was not going to be choosy. I was so grateful to hear that he was going to operate. That three months of waiting was very hard because my hip had deteriorated in that time."

In her suburb she had a choice of hospitals, because the surgeon operated at three different public hospitals.

She told the surgeon that she had an orthotic to compensate for the 5 cm (2 in) discrepancy in the length of her legs. He said he would see what could be done about that. She didn't take much notice of his remark at the time, because all she wanted was a new hip.

She thought that she might have to go into a **rehabilitation centre** to be looked after instead of continuing to live in her own apartment. Her decision was complicated by learning that the anti-inflammatory drug she was using tended to raise her blood pressure. She heard stories from other patients that were far from supportive of surgery. She became quite anxious.

> "It was really most disturbing. One little lady had to have hers redone because it wasn't done properly. I swallowed hard. I really was frightened, because I thought my foot deformity might be against me. A friend of mine has got brittle bones, and told me that it doesn't matter if the surgeon is good. 'It's your bones that count.' She fell — it wasn't arthritis in her case — and broke her hip. They put a plate in, and it worked loose, and she's had it done I think three times."

To add to her anxiety she heard about a man in his sixties who played a very good game of croquet. His hip became so bad that he couldn't walk, even with a stick. The doctor would not do an operation on his hip because he said he was too young.

> "They say the new hip lasts twenty years. This was a wicked thing to tell him, because that man has died since of something else. He shouldn't have had to suffer as he did."

Charles

While he had been in politics Charles had learned much about his state's hospitals. He made further, more personal, enquires about hospitals when the time came for him to have the hip operation, and he concluded that the best place was the same private hospital that had been recommended to me. He asked his physician to give him some names of surgeons who operated there. He chose a surgeon whom he had seen about a painful shoulder.

Charles's decision was affected by the seriousness of the operation, difficulties he had in getting about, his discomfort and pain, the risk of failure, assurances from relatives and friends, his age, and, finally, his interest in sport.

> "Anybody who takes on elective surgery very lightly is a mug. It is a very, very high-risk venture. You've really got to need it. The main reason I elected to have it was because of the considerable disability in moving around. I really was a mess on stairs. The limp was becoming pronounced, and a couple of friends said that if you let the limp get too bad, when you correct it you'll find it's still there. I think I've still got it anyway;

I probably did let it go a bit too long. A barrister mate of mine, who's a bit fat, still has a very bad limp ten years after getting his hip done. His colleagues say that he let it go too long. The doctors like to do it after the age of 60, not before. Or 45, when you get two in a lifetime."

Charles talked with friends, colleagues, and his son-in-law, who is a doctor, about the operation. His son-in-law assured him that the technology of the operation was continually improving and that the cement used was getting better. The surgeon showed Charles the prosthesis that lay on his desk.

"I talked with one of my colleagues, a friend, who's had both hips done. He had the second one done before I had my first, and he was in pretty bad shape, limping very badly before. His walk changed."

Charles loves cricket and football, so he decided to have the operation in April that year.

"I picked that time because the Australian cricketers were playing in England and the football was on. So I saw those great Australian innings at two in the morning. I wouldn't have seen them otherwise."

Doug

Doug was advised by orthopaedic surgeons at his university that good work was done at a private hospital not far from his home. One of the surgeons there, a particularly notable doctor, came highly recommended. So Doug went back to the medical centre at his university and got a referral to see the surgeon. At the same time he increased his private medical insurance and decided to have the operation in twelve months.

Not long before the operation he became anxious. He feared surgery, and considered seriously that he might put off the operation for another six months. But with only three months to go he had had enough pain.

"The last three months were the most difficult. I didn't take anything for the pain. I can't take anti-inflammatories because of the side effects. Also, I am a born coward, and the consequences of the surgery were quite frightening to me. I had had no surgery before, only tonsils. But as the pain increased, as my twelve months came to an end, I knew I was ready to go. No one tried to advise me to wait longer."

Ernst

Ernst saw his surgeon, a personal friend, on the advice of a sporting colleague, a specialist in sports medicine, who had long ago diagnosed arthritis of both hips in Ernst and suggested changes to his training methods. The surgeon confirmed the diagnosis and advised that nothing be done except to cease running. Ernst modified his training program by doing weightlifting while seated, saw the surgeon once a year, and gradually increased the use of anti-inflammatories, taking care to avoid interference to his digestion. He knew that many arthritis sufferers experience **nausea** and stomach pains if they take certain anti-inflammatory tablets. For that reason a doctor's prescription is needed to ensure that the tablets chosen do not have this unpleasant side effect. He increased the dose of his tablets on competition days and used extra painkiller. The pain got worse as the years passed.

After three years his surgeon proposed that the pain could be managed with an **osteotomy,** an operation in which the bone is cut in two and joined again at a slightly different angle. But Ernst continued as he was. Four years later he was using four anti-inflammatories and eight painkillers each day and finding his activities still curtailed.

"I couldn't confidently surf because being thrown about by the waves would cause pain, gardening was becoming a problem, and for about six years I'd sleep only on my back, my knees propped up with a pillow, with painkillers through the night."

He couldn't work effectively as a psychiatrist because he wasn't sleeping. So eventually the decision was made.

By now an osteotomy was out of the question; the only option was hip replacement. His surgeon watched Ernst as took his clothes off for the examination and put them on again, and said it might be better to wait another six months. Ernst did not agree.

"I wanted to recuperate while the Olympics were on. I always take two weeks off work every Olympics to watch them on television."

The decision to have them done immediately had the support of the retired sporting colleague whose advice Ernst had followed years before.

"The chap who used to coach me in hammer throwing — a doctor who lives in Spain now and has had his hips replaced too — wrote and said that with any luck the hip replacement will last twenty years. 'You're 45. Why don't you have them done now? Have them done again at 65. You should be dead by the time you need them done again.' I thought that made sense."

Ernst knew a major risk in the operation was from **deep vein thrombosis** in the leg. He had learned that in the 1960s up to 60 per cent of patients were getting deep vein thrombosis in the legs, and a significant percentage of those would get **pulmonary embolus** (a blood clot in the lung), which can be fatal. His surgeon advised him of more recent research.

"Now the incidence of deep vein thrombosis is reduced to between 1 and 3 per cent. As I understand it, wearing the white **TED/DVT stockings** has clear benefits. I'd be all for wearing them even if they're inconvenient and annoying. It stops the blood pooling in the lower leg. And if you get pooling you get stasis, the blood stops flowing, and then it clots. But it seems, from what my surgeon said to me, and from my medical training, that if you're relatively active you're less prone to getting deep vein thrombosis."

The white stockings are named TED/DVT full-length stockings. Some surgeons insist on patients wearing them in the belief that they help to prevent blood clotting in the deep veins of the lower leg, and thereby offset the serious problem of having a blood clot reach the lungs, which could be fatal.

His surgeon preferred to do **cementless** hip replacement in patients younger than 75 because it is much easier to do **revision surgery** (an operation on a hip that has already been replaced at least once) on a cementless hip than on a cemented one. Within ten years about 15 per cent of new hips either wear or become infected and might need to be replaced.

Ernst's decision was influenced by his athletic pastimes, and much control was in his hands. Ernst had two hammer-throwing championships early in the year, so he decided to have his operation a week after the second. His surgeon respected his personal views and capacity to decide. He said he did not need to see Ernst until his pain was unbearable, which it was by mid year.

Fred

Before Fred decided whether to have his operation he went to the medical library at a local university for recent books and articles on hip replacement. He discovered the different kinds of material used in prosthesis and whether they were cemented into the femur, and noted risks involved as well as the rates of success. Armed with this information, he questioned his surgeon closely and found him willing to answer. The surgeon was apparently pleased to have a patient so informed and interested in the technical procedures of the operation. Ever cautious, Fred found another surgeon and approached him in the same way. The second surgeon pushed Fred's questions aside.

"He was into the medical model. Keep them ignorant. Don't tell the patient a thing. I kept at him, and when I'd finished, I told him I didn't think much of his answers and that I wouldn't be back."

Helen

Altogether Helen had six hip operations about three years apart, and learned very little from her surgeon about what happened. She felt he had little time for her, and showed her little or no consideration, both at his surgery and in hospital.

"Some operations were just resurfacing; in others they reconstructed the hip entirely with a prosthesis and they made up a little ball. My surgeon doesn't believe in telling you much. He's of the old school. I've known him a long time. I said to him this morning, 'It is my body, you know.' He just looked at me. He doesn't believe in physiotherapists. When I went to see him last time he said in his quick snappy tone, 'Right, you can start putting weight on it; you can go like this.' He would come in, say, 'Right, no rolling on the other side for eight weeks; no weight on it for ten weeks; pillow between the legs when you sleep', and then another lot of instructions. He didn't even say goodbye. He'll be retiring probably next year or the year after. His partner, who is being groomed to take over, is the exact opposite. I saw him a couple of days ago. He seems very nice. He actually talks to you. The nurses tell you more than the surgeons do."

Mario

Mario was most anxious until one day he heard the surgeon talking to a student who had been assigned to him.

"I have a chronic blood disorder, haemochromatosis. It's quite likely that the blood disorder had contributed to the hip problem. The second surgeon had had experience with haemochromatosis. I felt more confident about him. I was most reassured because this surgeon was also a training surgeon, and he asked my permission to have a student present while he examined me. The advantage was that I could hear what they were talking about. I could learn something about it. While still having some apprehension about the operation I felt a lot better."

Many elderly customers at Mario's restaurant would ask him why he was limping. Then they would tell him what they knew about acquaintances of theirs who had had hips replaced. In this way Mario learned more and felt a little more secure in his decision.

The surgeon told him little. Mario was frightened, and glad that nothing more was said.

"I always call the prosthesis a honeycomb. It has that ability to fuse to the bone and the bone fuses to it. Cementless. He said there would be a longer recovery period because of the bone regrowth. He didn't go into a lot of detail about the operation, nor did I seek a lot of information. I didn't want to know what the process was. It's his business. I felt I could trust the surgeon."

Nell

Nell had her pain in the groin, and her general practitioner's assistant said that, from observing the way she moved, it was definitely a hip problem. He didn't require X-rays. He asked her to say when she could cope with pain no longer and then have the X-rays. He suggested she do exercises to build up the muscles. Nevertheless, when she saw her surgeon he did not agree with the advice on exercises, and suggested that exercises would only aggravate the hip because, in her case, there was nothing between the head of her femur and its socket. Her surgeon showed her the X-rays and described the operation.

> "The prosthesis was metal and put in with cement. I think it had a ceramic head and a sort of a plastic shield. He had a model on the desk. He described it all very well. Before I went to hospital, his nurse went through it in great detail, and all the financial side of it, how much I would get back, what he would charge. They were very good like that."

Her decision was based on what she could see quite clearly from the X-rays two months before the operation.

> "I made the date, really. I just couldn't put up with the pain any longer. It wasn't only when I was walking. I couldn't even get comfortable lying flat in bed, and it was painful putting on shoes."

Sonomi

Sonomi's rheumatologist said she needed a new hip. She went on a search for the right surgeon. She saw three. The one Sonomi chose warned her about the risk of blood clotting and infection, and reassured her that the hospital he used admitted few patients for long-term treatment and consequently was less likely than many others to harbour infections. Dislocation was always a possibility, he told her, but it was very rare because of the excellent nursing at that hospital. He advised her to make two **autologous blood donations**, and since she was well insured the maximum cost to her would be modest. She chose that surgeon because he was the most considerate of the three.

Tess

Tess's trouble appeared in originally 1983. She had tried physio-therapy, but the pain persisted. Her surgeon advised her that the new hip would last about seven years.

> "They wanted you well over 80 so that you probably wouldn't need another one. That was why, when I first went to see my surgeon, he said, 'I don't think we want to do that yet. I think you're too young to have it done yet.' In the end I went to see him on a Thursday, and he made up his mind and said: 'I can do you on Tuesday if you like.' I was amazed and asked: 'Can I have it done on Tuesday?' 'Of course. It's got to be done.' So I didn't have any time to worry. He was one of the best to do it. And I went in very happily. I was happy to be able to walk properly and to do things again."

Her second hip operation, a revision, arose from pain, high hopes, and the fact that she was in good health for her age.

> "My surgeon thought he would change it again. I was well and healthy, and he thought I would stand the operation. I expected to come out and go through the same procedure, and it would be the same as the first one. 'I'll put you back to the original.' So I said, 'Right.' I was quite thrilled to be going in again. For the same hip."

Wendy

Wendy was also advised to delay the operation and to relieve pain by using a walking stick. She did, but returned in a few years com-plaining that her quality of life was poor. And she was fed up with the pain. The surgeon wanted her to keep waiting and suggested drilling a few holes in the femur to help regain some of the lost blood supply in the head of the femur. This procedure would delay the hip operation, which at that time was thought to be effective for only ten to fifteen years. Since Wendy was in her thirties, she would probably need several new hips in her lifetime.

Disconcerted by this prospect, she discussed the surgeon's advice with her general practitioner, who then suggested getting another opinion. The second surgeon said that, because Wendy's injury was so old, the drilling would not help regain enough blood to make such a procedure worthwhile. Instead he suggested that every year she delayed was a bonus. So she delayed for five years. He advised her that once the pain started waking her at night, she ought not tolerate it any more.

Wendy's brother, a general practitioner, sent her information from a medical journal on hip replacements. She found it gruesome to look at, but discussions with her surgeon had prepared her.

In the last couple of years the surgeon told her of the new prosthesis, which was covered with porous material, looked like a honeycomb, and bonded itself to the bone instead of being secured with cement.

(3)

Becoming a patient

In a private health system it is usual to have the hip replacement operation within about five weeks, largely because this allows enough time for the surgeon, the hospital, and the patient to prepare for the operation. In that five weeks I had to do many things: prepare myself physically and medically for the operation; attend the hospital shortly before the operation to discover what would be going on when I was admitted; gather items to take to hospital; make plans for my one-month recovery period at home, or in a rehabilitation centre, after leaving hospital; and finally I had to pay for all this.

The cost of the operation

I had decided to have the operation at the private hospital where my surgeon worked regularly. I was fully insured, and the surgeon's nurse–secretary showed me a list of the costs, including the surgeon's fees and estimates of fees charged by the anaesthetist, the surgeon's assistant and other colleagues, for example, the consultant physician, the **radiologist** who took X-rays, and the **pathologist** who tested blood. Altogether I would be out off pocket by a small amount.

Bernard also was fully insured, and felt that he was due for something in return for so many years' contributions.

"We've been paying private health insurance for years and not getting anything out of it. We worked it out. At the time it was going to cost us thousands without insurance. I think it did cost us about $500 with the insurance. The stainless steel hip thing alone was thousands."

Nell had a similar experience; Helen, a young student, was supported by her father.

"I've never really earned enough to be able to afford it, so he's always paid for it. He is now on the top insurance schedule. But three years ago when I had the right hip done, he'd just changed his insurance. He ended up having to pay about five or six grand."

The same held in 1983 for Tess, but then the surgeon rather than his nurse–secretary issued the warning.

"He said straight away to my husband, 'It's going to cost. It's an expensive operation, it's a big operation. I hope you're well insured.' My husband replied, 'We're in the top bracket.' 'Well, you'll be OK.' He chose the hospital. He worked there a lot."

Aware of the high cost, Doug delayed his operation for a year. For years he had paid health insurance premiums at an intermediate level of benefits, not the top level.

"I made a decision to fix my medical benefits from intermediate level to the top level. That meant I had to serve twelve months. You are not allowed to have a pre-existing condition. You have to allow a twelve-month qualifying period."

Fred had his operation in a public hospital because his research showed that public hospitals were better equipped to manage complications and emergencies during or after an operation. In his case the hospital fees themselves would have been lower than those in a private hospital. He paid top health insurance cover so he was free to choose his own surgeon, in a public hospital. Betty also used a public hospital.

"Everything was covered by insurance. I didn't pay a penny. Top private cover. If I had gone to a different hospital I might've had to pay. When I see the surgeon now, I still don't pay him. I pay for the X-rays and the blood tests I have."

The operation is regarded as elective surgery, because no matter how much pain you are in, a total hip replacement is not a matter of life and death.

If you are not insured and cannot afford the operation, you will have to go to a public hospital, where you will wait much longer than five weeks. One doctor told her patient that the wait was five years; a recent newspaper report said the wait was between six months and one year; one hospital authority told me recently that you could wait between three months and three years. So the waiting period at a public hospital for people without health insurance is highly variable.

To establish how variable, I asked at a large public hospital what were their policies and practices regarding total hip replacement for people who could not afford to pay. I was told that the decision to operate is based on medical factors and the patient's age and health. After the medical decision is made, the patient is put in a queue. The hospital aims to do the operation in between three and six months; this period could be affected when a patient has personal reasons for asking to delay the date of the operation. These days, on average the operation is actually done within a year. Rarely does a patient have to wait three years. This is so for most public hospitals.

In the public hospital system there is another point to consider. Not only would you have to wait a long time in pain for the operation but also you would have to recover in a ward of four to six beds. Further, the conditions for patients are less comfortable than in a private hospital, and the food is not as good. If these considerations matter to you, and your hip is in trouble, be advised to take out the best health insurance you can afford. Otherwise you pay an account of many thousands of dollars, or have a long wait in agony and an adequate but less comfortable recovery.

Reorganising your commitments

Your decision to have a new hip will affect many people, so as soon as you know when and where the operation is to be done, advise them how long you expect to be out of action. When I told my boss at the university, disarray followed because there was no provision to cover my teaching commitments for eight weeks, and those commitments had to be met. I was told I had to put my teaching on video and to find two people to present and discuss the work in class. This made my five weeks preparation very busy indeed.

To help the administration of sick leave it was necessary for me to get a statement from the surgeon saying how long he expected I would be unavailable for work. In the first instance he made it eight weeks, providing all went well and there were no complications. My surgeon would have advised another month's leave had problems arisen.

You might need to find out how long you can be away from work without being sacked or losing entitlements, for example, sick leave and leave without pay. If you have a desk job, plan to be away from it for eight weeks. Nevertheless, one of my colleagues was back in his office three weeks after the operation. He could not stand life at home with only daytime TV programs to occupy him! If you have a heavy job, negotiate to be assigned less strenuous tasks on your return to work.

Charles planned life with a new hip carefully. He had retired from politics and was working at a university.

"I was no longer in Parliament at that stage. I had prepared for the operation for four months. I culled my commitments at university and made other arrangements, and I really was not apprehensive about having to take three or four months. I knew it would be a long time."

Mario prepared himself according to the personal needs of his family. His main problem was to plan how the family restaurant business could cope with his absence, and to decide how the family could manage to help him during his long recovery period. Nell had a less complex situation.

"I work in a family business and I've been there for some years now. They just said to take off whatever you want."

Working commitments are not the only demands to be affected by the decision to have new hip. You won't be able to visit your elderly relatives, look after small children, or do housework for at least two weeks after you get back home. Pets will need feeding while you are away, and home deliveries will have to be cancelled. If you live alone you will need to find a sympathetic helper to care for you for at least a month after you leave hospital. If you have no such person, then plan to live in, or close to, a rehabilitation centre for at least two weeks. Hospital staff are the best people to advise on choosing a rehabilitation centre. If you do not go to such a centre, and you do not have a live-in helper, arrange for someone to visit you daily for at least two weeks.

In short, anticipate that you will be out of action for about two months, and maybe unable to carry out usual everyday activities for almost six. If you tell people this, they will make the necessary adjustments. If you do not, you might find they lack understanding and become unsympathetic during the slow stages of your recovery.

Choosing the right hospital

You can choose the hospital you want, but as a rule the surgeon will lead you to choose the hospital that he or she is most familiar with or is using regularly. Fred looked into private and public hospitals, and decided on a public hospital because he was convinced that public hospitals had better resources than private hospitals to meet any emergency.

Charles chose his surgeon, and the surgeon chose a private hospital, one that enjoyed a fine reputation and where many new hips had been implanted. Then a problem arose. About two weeks before his operation Charles was having a routine blood check at a public hospital when a man came up to him.

"He said, 'Mr —, you must know about this.' He thought I was still in politics, I think. He said, 'My wife is in this private hospital where you are going.' His story was that she'd been to the private hospital, had a hip replacement, and she got a very bad infection. She'd turned up as an emergency case at this public hospital where I was. They took her whole prosthesis out and started again. He even gave me the name of the surgeon. It's a terrible story. So I rang my surgeon and he said, 'Well, I'll find out about this.' He came back and assured me that the private hospital was terrific. I said, 'Well, you've all got golden staph in your hospitals, I know that, and you can't get it out. Is this private hospital better than most?' He said, 'Well, it's all right.' His story was that the patient was too fat, she hadn't done her exercises, and it was all her fault. That was the extent of my research about the hospital."

Medical check-up

Charles's story about infection and the overweight patient indicates that before the surgeon operates he or she needs to know
how healthy a patient you are. I was told to have a medical check-
up and to get a blood test. Further X-rays were taken once I had
been admitted to hospital a day before the operation. For me and
for Doug this was a most important part of the preparation because
of its effects on us personally.

I went to see a specialist in cardiology, a friend of more than
twenty years, who told me that I was very healthy and that I need
have no concerns about the operation. Strong heart. Sound lungs.
All the things I wanted to hear. I left the office in the highest of
spirits, pleased to be healthy enough to have this operation.
Nothing to fear. All he needed was for me to have a blood test and
ensure that the results were sent to him.

Doug too was healthy and pleased to be so.

"I had a complete pre-op examination. Blood, heart, lungs, all came up to
normal."

Bernard too had a medical check-up and found that he had a
little blood pressure, nothing more.

Improving your health

Is there something more that you can do about your health other
than be examined and given the OK?

Lose weight

When my surgeon introduced me to his nurse–secretary he left us
saying that I should lose a bit of weight. Later I discovered that it
was a good idea to be as light as possible before the operation so
as to reduce the stress on the new hip, and to ensure a secure and
speedy recovery. A kilo (about 2 lb) around the middle equals 3 kg
(about 6 lb) pressure on a hip. So I tried to reduce my weight by
eating less and dropping some fattening foods. If you are overweight consider seeing a dietitian who could help you to lose
weight without going on a faddish diet.

Charles remembered the story of the overweight woman.

"I took off a bit of weight, too. I just did it myself. I was never very heavy. I took off about a stone [14 lb; 6.5 kg]. I went from eleven stone, seven [161 lb; 73 kg] in the old measures down to about ten, seven [147 lb; 67 kg]."

Bernard's doctor suggested that he lose a bit of weight.

"... which I thought was a bit strange. All these years I've been trying to put a bit of weight on, not take it off. I had to have a high fibre diet. We do eat a lot of vegetables anyway so that didn't change."

On the other hand, Terri's doctor suggested that she not lose weight, which she felt was sensible.

"I was not under weight, but they said you need all your energy reserves."

Ernst dropped his weight because of what he had learned about a rare complication that might follow the hip replacement operation.

"I dropped my weight 7 kg [15. 5 lb] for the operation — and I'm still down in weight — because I used to keep my weight up deliberately for athletics purposes, and I have found heavier people are more prone to get **heterotopic ossification.**"

Medical research indicates that overweight patients are more likely to have this happen. Being a large man, Ernst was fearful of this complication after reading about hip replacements.

Exercise

For about a year before his operation Fred, who never needed to lose weight, had worked out in a gym and had been swimming regularly. He wanted the odds as much in his favour as possible. Charles did much the same for a shorter period.

"To prepare for the operation, I did some exercises the physio gave me. Tightening your buttocks and all that stuff. And the bike exercise was often good for it. I used to ride the bike about 15–20 km [9–12 miles] a day, three or four times a week."

The exercises Charles mentioned are available from a physiotherapist and are intended to strengthen your legs and muscles. They can be done night and morning, and whenever possible

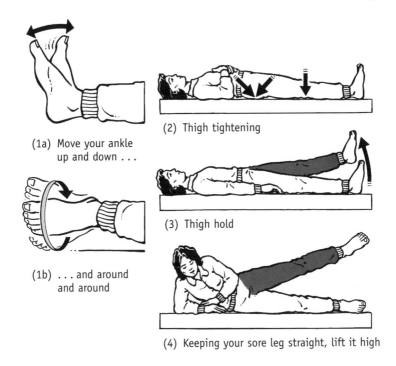

(1a) Move your ankle
up and down . . .

(1b) . . . and around
and around

(2) Thigh tightening

(3) Thigh hold

(4) Keeping your sore leg straight, lift it high

Figure 4: Four exercises to prepare you for the operation.

during the day. The first one is to move your ankles up, down and around. The second is to lie down flat on your back, press the back of your knees into the floor and, at the same time, tighten your thighs. Repeat this ten times. Third, lift one leg about 15 cm (6 in) off the floor, and count to five while you keep your leg straight. Do the other leg. Repeat the exercise ten times too. Fourth, lie on your good side and, keeping your bad leg straight, lift it as high as you can, count to five, then lower it. Try this five times.

Rather than riding the exercise bike vigorously, Charles could have exercised gently on a stationary bicycle, gone swimming, or done gentle stretching. For some people swimming might be out because getting into the pool might prove difficult; even so, pools for hydrotherapy are built with steps and rails for the disabled.

Because you will be in bed for ten days or more and must often pull yourself up, sit up, and push yourself around in the bed, it could be helpful to strengthen your stomach muscles. You will have a triangular steel device above your head, known as a 'monkey bar', to pull yourself off your bottom so you can be washed and otherwise cared for. It would be helpful if your arm muscles were up to the task. Strong arms are a help in bed, especially when one leg is in pain and weak. Strong arms are also useful for using crutches when you begin to walk shortly after the operation. A physiotherapist can help you with the appropriate exercises, or you could go to a gym and get help if you tell the trainer exactly what you need. Of course you cannot regain the strength you enjoyed when young, but exercise and weight control for the five weeks before the operation could help your recovery.

Being an athlete and a doctor, Ernst knew that exercising his body would help him control pain after surgery.

"I was worried about pain control for the first operation, and I spoke to an anaesthetist. I prepared for it by training three to five times a week, weight training and exercise bikes. I was cardiovascularly fit, and I had very strong bone stock, because of all the weightlifting. I'm very strong in the legs, and I think that is what gave me a big advantage."

Some candidates for a new hip are very healthy because of their lifestyle. Young housewives and mothers like Wendy are a good examples. She looked after a household of seven, thrived at home and waited many years before she was old enough to have a new hip.

"I didn't do anything, no exercises or physiotherapy. My biggest problem was time, really. I had five young kids."

For some people exercise is not appropriate or necessary. Helen, an unusual case, suffers badly from juvenile rheumatoid arthritis. She had undergone several operations in the last five years. She followed her surgeon's advice not to undertake physiotherapy without his close supervision.

"I'm very cautious about my diet, and made sure that it was very good, and I also wrote down my diet for ten days and went to see a dietitian before I went in to see if I was on the right track. I don't eat many dairy products, and I was always a bit worried about my calcium levels. I also did a lot of walking beforehand because I wanted to strengthen the right leg. The left's always been my good leg; the right's always been a bit weak, so I thought I'd better strengthen it. My surgeon was very anti-physio, he doesn't believe in physios."

Smoking

Changing your environment and radically altering your everyday behaviour and habits, which you are forced to do when becoming a candidate for a new hip, is a good opportunity to give up smoking. Many people find they can give it up when they go to hospital because no one is allowed to smoke there, and because the shock to their body is so great that a cigarette is the last thing they want.

Smoking can endanger your recovery. Why? During an operation a smoker is more likely to stop breathing than a non-smoker, and some smokers stop breathing after the operation when they need oxygen to recover. If you smoke, now is the chance to quit, to convince yourself that smoking is not a sensible way of managing your feelings and problems in everyday life, and to adopt healthier and more effective ways of coping. Try to quit at least two weeks before the operation if you can't do it now.

If fear of breathtaking complications is not enough to motivate you to stop, ask the Anti-Cancer Council or a similar organisation in your state for a brochure with helpful hints on how to quit smoking. You might even consider therapy, like hypnosis, from a psychologist.

Your blood or theirs?

During a hip operation and for a while afterwards you could lose between 1 and 2.5 litres (2–4 pints) of blood. Usually people lose about a half a litre (1 pint), but since the operation is not entirely predictable it is necessary to have a supply of blood on hand in case of emergencies.

My surgeon said he would like me to put aside my own blood for the operation rather than use blood from a blood bank. Using your own blood ensures that you are not risking infection. Even though all blood in the blood bank is carefully tested with advanced techniques of blood analysis, it is possible that there might be a new blood disease that has yet to be established or a new virus that has not been discovered. So the advice now is to use your own blood. You do this by making an autologous (relating to the self) blood donation to a blood bank, which makes your blood available to the hospital shortly before your operation.

In the last three weeks before the operation I was scheduled to give three units of 450 ml (almost a pint) each. After the second unit I was told that a third would not be necessary. The standard is two units. Later I found that although three units is the commonly scheduled number of units, surgeons rarely need that much blood to replace what is lost in a hip operation. Also I learned that the third unit would have been donated to a blood bank for use by another patient had it not been used by my surgeon at the time of my operation.

Today I am still unsure about how much blood is needed for the hip operation and whether it is, or can be, saved for use by others if not used by me. The experience of other informants was equally unclear, except Ernst who, after the operation, managed to obtain his unused blood to hasten his recovery. Doug gave his own blood beforehand, and he said the amount was 2 litres in two bags. Charles went down to the local public hospital to give blood, four lots of blood, 800 ml at a time, or so he thought!

"I gave four blood donations. He insisted on four. Eight hundred millilitres — does that sound right? I didn't like giving blood, and I used to come away feeling a bit nauseous; not really sick, though. That had to be done within a month, because the first one is no good if it is older than thirty-one days. I had a good **blood count**, I think it was 16.5 [i.e. 16.5 g per 100 ml of blood]. I think normal is 12. I did have to take **iron tablets** because my blood count went down so rapidly. By the time I gave the last autologous blood donation it was down to about 11, I think."

A blood count involves counting the number of red and white cells in a known amount of blood. From the blood count of red cells an estimate is made of the **haemoglobin** in the bloodstream. Haemoglobin determines the efficiency with which the bloodstream carries oxygen through the body to maintain its tissues. It takes up oxygen as blood passes through the lungs and releases it as blood passes through the tissues. Normally the haemoglobin level is 12–18 g per 100 ml of blood in men and 11–15 g per 100 ml in women. In hospital a patient's haemoglobin level — often itself called a 'blood count' — is estimated regularly by taking samples of blood. After the shock of surgery the level varies from patient to patient and for each patient from time to time.

For this reason it is vital to monitor the blood to know whether sufficient oxygen is available to help damaged tissues heal. If the 'blood count' falls unexpectedly to unacceptable levels, the patient could be given a transfusion of blood to bring the 'blood count' into the normal range and thereby maintain the rate of recovery.

Bernard was put on iron tablets and vitamin C. He decided to use his own blood. Again, the amount varied.

"It took a unit a week over a month. Four units were taken to be on the safe side. They only used one in the finish. The number that they suggested was normal. That didn't worry me at all."

Ernst planned the autologous blood donations carefully and put himself on iron supplements and vitamin C to aid the absorption of iron in food. Nell gave blood several times beforehand.

"It was the simplest thing in the world, I found. Perfectly all right. I hadn't given blood before at all, but it was no problem at all. They give you a nice cup of tea and a sandwich afterwards. It was quite pleasant. I went to a local public hospital three times to give blood, once a week I think. I was taking some iron tablets. They said to take them, and I did and I didn't. I wasn't awfully good about that. I forgot."

Tess said that for her first hip operation there was no suggestion of putting aside her own blood.

"In those days you went straight in, and they gave you whatever blood they had. They didn't talk about autologous blood in those days."

For her second operation it was too much trouble to go to the blood bank to donate the blood. She could do it in the hospital itself just before the operation.

For two of my informants, giving blood raised a problem. Betty did not want to donate her own blood, and she had her own reasons.

"I was asked, 'Do you want to give your own blood?' and I said, 'No.' I used to give blood during the Second World War, but I'm too old now to give blood, and with my blood pressure I wasn't prepared to offer to give blood. I think I would've been advised against giving it. If it was an accident in the street I'd have to take a risk with someone else's blood. So I just had the blood bank blood."

Mario was a unusual case, too. He suffered from haemachromotosis (too much iron in the blood), so it was necessary to draw off a litre of blood every three months. He made an autologous blood donation of three bags.

> "It's something that you never quite get used to, people sticking things in you and taking blood away. It was just a nuisance. I went to the blood bank, because the blood is treated there."

The amount of blood needed seems to vary with the surgeon and the patient. At least two and no more than four units of 450 ml (almost a pint) are sought. But three things are clear: an iron supplement might be needed to replace the iron that is lost when blood is donated; iron-rich food, such as spinach, nuts, and red meat, is probably the right thing to eat at the time; and at meal times a vitamin C tablet could be taken to help you absorb the iron from the food.

Ceasing the anti-inflammatories

The surgeon's nurse–secretary had told me that about ten days before the operation I should stop taking my anti-inflammatory tablets. Later I learned that, like aspirin, the tablets thin the blood. During the operation and in recovery it would make me susceptible to bleeding freely. When I did stop taking the tablets my hip was in great pain. I phoned her. She said I could take special painkillers available at the pharmacy without prescription. That was fine.

Charles had the same experience, but handled it differently.

> "I was just told not, under any circumstances, to take any of those anti-inflammatories. And I took nothing for the pain."

For Nell the decision did not seem to matter.

> "They may've said to stop taking anti-inflammatory tablets, and I think I just went on as normal and went into hospital and had it done."

Ernst had doubts about the advice and the reason for following it. The problem was related to his family history, not the difficulties at the time of the operation.

"I had to give up the anti-inflammatories because my father had had a clotting problem when operated on by the same surgeon. He was a bit wary and, instead of the usual two weeks before the operation, he said to stop taking them three weeks before. Well, that really wreaked havoc with me because I seized up. Although I was still able to win the championships, my performance dropped dramatically because I couldn't move my hips. I had terrible problems, so I had to increase the painkillers, to take on much stronger ones, just to get through the day with no anti-inflammatories. One of the medical articles I read says very clearly that anti-inflammatories only really need to be stopped one day before the operation, even though the conventional advice is two weeks."

Whether it is one day, ten days or two weeks before the operation, it is necessary to cease taking the anti-inflammatories. For sound advice ask your surgeon. A stronger drug could be taken if the pain is great when the anti-inflammatories are cut out. Furthermore, some doctors advise female patients who take other drugs that seriously affect their hormone functioning, such as oral contraceptive pills or hormone replacement therapy, to stop some weeks before the operation. Again, all advice on taking drugs is best sought from your surgeon or doctor.

Plans for your return home

Before my operation I spent at least two days alone, mooching about the house, and getting it clean for the time when I would return.

What should I do about having a shower and using the lavatory? Years ago I had connected an outside hot shower for the children after they had come back from the beach. I thought that would be the best way to have a shower. I had planned to rent a chair that fitted over the lavatory seat when I came home from hospital. I did not think about other matters. Now I would advise people who are living alone to make a list for their return home, whether or not someone will be living in to care for you during the four-week recovery period.

In preparation for the operation and coming home Betty, a widow, told her general practitioner that she lived alone in an apartment, had to approach it up thirty-two steps, and wondered whether the effort would be too much for her immediately after the operation. Should she live elsewhere? Should she sell her apartment? The doctor advised her to stay put and showed no concern about the stairs. People came from the hospital to see where she lived and, after assessing her home, sent workmen to install rails in the bathroom and toilet.

"I didn't pay for the jobs. That's how caring they were at the hospital."

Hospital staff said she would need physiotherapy after the operation and asked her who would be at the apartment when she returned from hospital. They gave her a brochure telling about the physiotherapist's exercises before she went to hospital, and gave her another copy when she went home. She agreed to go to physiotherapy and attend a rehabilitation centre for a short period, and arranged for a friend to come and stay with her for three months.

Wendy was not alone. She had a husband and five young children.

"I had to pace myself. I used to sit down a fair bit, for ironing or peeling vegetables, and I had a very supportive husband. He really is terrific, and I did get a lady to do the main housework, like the floors. I could just do the other bits of housework, washing and ironing."

Careful planning for the return home is needed, because you cannot bend through more than 90 degrees, and, without the support of walking aids, you could very easily topple and not be able to get up without pain. Being unable to drive a car for six weeks or more means someone else will have to shop for you, or you will have to shop by phone and get things delivered. And you must remember to ask the delivery person to bring the items into the house, not drop them at the front door, and put them on a bench, not the floor, so you can reach them. If you like watching television and using your VCR, be sure it is at table height.

Being unable to bend is not only frustrating and infuriating, it can also be disastrous. If you bend down quickly to catch a ball of wool, a spoon, or a magazine that has fallen from your lap, you might find yourself back in hospital with a dislocated hip. Grabbing or reaching for the soap when it slips to the bathroom floor is another dangerous action. If you twist too quickly while using the toilet, either to clean yourself or to get at the toilet paper the same could happen. When going to the toilet tear off the paper first, then be cautious, be slow, and avoid extending yourself. Forget the wool and the magazine, or use an **extension arm** to retrieve it. Buy a spare cake of soap, and a soap on a rope.

It is worth repeating: if you live alone make a list of what you do before you go to the hospital. Ask the hospital to help you find an **occupational therapist** to visit you and go through the list. Show the occupational therapist what you normally do around the house. Then follow their professional advice for your unique circumstances. If you do not live alone, talk with the person who will be helping you, and agree on how you might live for the four weeks or more of recovery.

An excellent source of advice is another person who has recently had a new hip. Bernard had a neighbour who had got a new hip two years earlier and lent him her toilet chair, crutches, walking stick, extension arm and the sock-aid for putting socks on without help.

Kitchen and laundry

Give up using the dishwasher; instead put a dish drainer on the sink and keep the cleaning brush and detergent near by. You won't be able to get at any items beneath the sink for a week or so. Frozen food in a refrigerator with a bottom freezing unit is out. Saucepans under the kitchen bench, washing liquid or powder under the washing trough, or a front-loading washing machine should all be ignored. It is hard to get into a top-loading washing machine without an extension arm.

If you live alone all these items will have to be at table height or within reach above, or left to someone else to manage. You will need a clothes horse to hang your washing on, and it should be placed high so that you can use the lower rungs. An electric clothes dryer will be a problem unless you can raise it on a small table or bench in the laundry.

Putting so many things on the benches in the kitchen will limit your work space at waist level. You might like to buy or borrow a trolley or an auto tray, or perhaps convert the laundry cart into a temporary trolley so that you can put on it items that seem to be in the way, and which you might need again soon.

How do you organise your refrigerator and dry foods? Buy in the food you use regularly and place it where you can reach it easily without stretching or bending down. If you put the smaller items in plastic bags with the handles facing you as you close the cupboard, you could use a shelf a little lower than waist height. Plan to use a microwave oven for cooking; but if you want to cook on a stove, put the saucepans on the stove or at stove-top height. Use only small or medium-sized saucepans, because large one will be heavy to lift when full. Put the lighter glasses a little higher, and make space for the heavier dishes and plates at waist level.

Clothes storage

You will need to think about your clothes and how they are stored at home. I kept my underwear and socks in two draws at chest height. I should have hung my shirts and sweaters in the wardrobe instead of keeping them in low drawers.

Gardening

I do little in the garden except basic maintenance. No longer could I mow the grass. Someone came to do that regularly through the summer. Digging was painful. Stooping was difficult. Now I can see that if you want to be a gardener it is best to get long-handled tools, and be prepared to let the garden go for some time after you recover. The best gardening advice would come from a garden fanatic who has already had a new hip put in.

Bedding

Your bed might be too low. Because I am tall I reckoned that if I put a futon between the mattress and the bed base, the bed would be raised enough for my comfort. I was right. But not everyone has a spare futon. There are special fittings made to raise your bed, and they are available from shops that cater for disabled people. Ask the occupational therapist at the hospital, or visit the nearest **Independent Living Centre**, or a similar organisation, where you can see everything that can be used to make living at home easier when you are disabled.

Seating

Your chairs around the house might be too low. I had four old bar stools with backs. Today you would find such chairs only at a charity shop or a second-hand furniture store. Also I had a carver, an old chair with arms, and a similar dining chair. These two chairs with arms and the bar stool were dotted about the house so I could sit anywhere when I felt the need.

Bathroom and toilet

Your toilet will be too low. On the day I was discharged I rented a seat like the one used in hospital, and so did all my informants. The height of the toilet seat can be adjusted to suit you.

Having a shower will be difficult, but by the time you get home you will have trained yourself to be cautious and slow in slippery places like the bathroom. Your bathroom might need special attention. On the slippery floor in the bath or shower recess, you can either use a bath mat or attach anti-slip strips available from a hardware store. In the shower you might benefit from a plastic shower chair like the chair you will use over the toilet seat in hospital. I showered outside with a garden shower that had been attached to an external extension to the hot water. The weather was warm enough for showering outdoors. I found that after a week I could use the shower over the bath because I was recovering well and had supports to grip while lifting my operated leg into the bath and on to a bath mat.

To make showering easier you can ask for an occupational therapist to help you work out how to use your bathroom. Where will you put your crutches while having a shower? And the extension arm? Should you use rubber mats or strips in the shower or bath? Rubber mats must be picked up, dried, and cleaned regularly. Who will do that? Maybe a hand shower extension should be installed. Probably you would use it in future, for washing your hair. Soap on a rope or in a soap holder? Soap on a rope can be made by putting the cake into one leg of a pair of pantyhose. Liquid soap instead of a cake? Shampoo in the holder too? Where should the holder be suspended from? Will you clean your feet with a long-handled brush? How will that hang up so that it is within reach?

If the bathroom has a drain in the floor, you could sit in a plastic chair and use an extension to the shower or basin tap to wash yourself by hand while seated.

Useful items to take to hospital

You will probably need to take all your medical identification items. I did not. Fortunately I had given the administration all the information they needed at a pre-admission clinic. But many hospitals do not have such arrangements. The medical identification data include X-rays, CT scans, blood type, hospital insurance information, list of medications and health problems, and your official medical card.

I made a list of items to take to hospital from advice in a brochure that the surgeon's nurse gave me. The list included a shoehorn with a long handle, little moist paper towels for wiping one's hands clean, paper tissues, soap on a rope, and night attire. I chose nightshirts, which I had been given by my neighbour. Be warned: nightshirts that reach far beyond your knee might be so long that they catch in your crutches when you are learning to walk. Shortie pyjamas seem best for both men and women.

On my feet I wore thick-soled shoes without laces that were secured by Velcro tabs across the top of the foot. Bernard used the same, and we both agreed they were the best items we took to hospital. They also made dressing easy when we came home. I wore no socks in hospital because I had to wear TED/DVT white stockings.

I took talcum powder, toothpaste, a comb and a hairbrush, an electric razor, and a couple of pairs of underpants. A friend lent me an extension arm and piece of sheepskin to put under me while in bed to help prevent bed rash. These days more hospitals are providing the sheepskin.

Other people recommend taking a little money for newspapers and chemist items; I found these could be put on the hospital account. Some hospitals give you a daily paper.

The hospital supplied me with elbow crutches and paper tissues. I had no use for the shoehorn because the shoes I used with

Velcro tabs could be taken on and off with the extension arm. Be warned: do not use scuffs or enclosed slippers on your feet. They are a hazard when using crutches. I never saw or used a sock aid, but some informants swear by them. The nurses showed me how a helper could put on socks and the TED/DVT stockings with a small plastic bag. For me the moist paper towels were unnecessary. From the hospital chemist I had to get a special talcum powder for the rash I developed on my back.

Before his operation, Ernst prepared himself with similar items.

"I got an extension arm and a long-handled shoehorn. I used them both. I still use the shoehorn when I'm putting on my golf shoes because they're hard to put on. And I got a sock aid to help me put socks on. I'd thread the sock over the sock aid and then put my foot in it and then pull it up with strings. I had a stool for in the shower, a high chair with arms, and I had a toilet booster seat, a round bubble one."

Betty had similar items and invented one of her own.

"I had a pick-up stick [extension arm]. It was invaluable. They provided me with that before the operation. I bought myself one. I made myself the soap on a rope, because its use depends on how tall you are. They only have a short cord. I took a bit of cord, and I put a hole in a piece of soap. You don't need to buy one. I made a sponge on a rope, too, because you can't afford to drop it. I like to get down and put the soap on my feet. I actually made several of those to give to people who subsequently had hip operations."

There is no point in renting personal items before you use them in the hospital. A kind friend lent me his underarm crutches, but they were too short for me, and the surgeon required me to use elbow crutches. The first pair were sent to me from the hospital pharmacy, and they too did not extend far enough for my height. Also my friend lent me a walking stick, and it too was short. I bought one from the shop at the hospital on the day I was discharged and used it for several weeks. Some months later I saw many different walking sticks and extension arms in shops that cater for the disabled. New models seem to be released regularly.

The pre-admission clinic

The pre-admission clinic was most interesting and did much to relieve me of the anxiety that naturally precedes an operation. I was the only person at this clinic; usually there are several patients. Two nurses took my medical history, weighed me and measured my legs, and took my blood pressure. I was shown into a room, prepared like the private room I would have in the hospital. I sat on the bed, saw how it worked and how I could lift myself up with a steel triangle, or monkey bar, just in reach above my head, and felt the large, firm, triangular pillow, an abduction pillow also known as a **Charnley pillow**, which would be strapped to my ankles after the operation.

At first I would be lying on my back, or be half inclined; after a day or so I would be walking about with a frame, then with a pair of crutches, then only one crutch, and finally with a walking stick or one crutch, depending on what the surgeon advised. I would have a raised seat to use in the toilet; I would be sitting on a chair to shower myself for a few days after the operation, and perhaps after a few days I would be walking the corridors of the ward. I was much cheered and comforted by this information and the opportunity to become familiar with the items that would be with me when I awoke.

One nurse checked my personal details again, then she said something that really pleased me. She asked me for my surgeon's name, and muttered, 'He's the best.' This was most reassuring. What better news could an anxious patient hear the day before the operation?

From the pre-admission clinic Bernard was grateful to learn how he would be helped to walk by a physiotherapist after the operation and how to use the toilet.

"We had a day where we went to the hospital before the operation. The wife went along with me, and we thought it was very good. There were three or four of us having the operation. The medical staff talked about the general things which were going to happen. We met the physio and the nurse, and we saw the bed go up and down, and they did show you the toilet seat that you might have to use. It's just not normal, is it? Especially when you're lying flat on your back."

At the clinic Ernst saw a video of an interview.

"He gave me this video, which explains the situation. It is an interview with a lady who's had a hip replaced, and her husband. They talk about the whole experience of going through it. One of the things I was very positive about was the pre-admission visit. They measure you for the TED/DVT stockings. Show you the Charnley pillow. A little medical history is taken, and people who will look after me turn up. That's nice."

On the other hand, Doug was relatively unprepared for what would happen at the hospital. He had booked in months beforehand, and there was no pre-admission clinic.

"Show you the bed? You've got to be joking. It was a big surprise to me. Show you the pillow you have between your legs? No. They sent me out information, and some, showing three different types of hips, was given to me when I went to see the surgeon. The introduction into the hospital could've been better. Or the standard literature they gave you could have given you tips about hospital life. I knew the triangular support above was available over the bed."

Mario also found there was no pre-admission clinic that he could attend, but he felt that he was well prepared. Terri read what to expect.

"I had read a book on this woman who had had a hip replacement. It came from the Arthritis Foundation. I don't think she really went into the procedures at hospital. It was what to expect when you get home, what you can or can't do."

In Wendy's nursing days, total hip replacements did not exist.

"They did a thing called a **Moore's prosthesis**. And that was pretty innovative in those days. But I didn't ever see any of that sort of thing. Mostly older people would fracture the femur, and they would put a plate in."

Moore's prosthesis was an early procedure that involved replacing only the head of the femur and not the socket of the acetabulum.

Later Wendy did obtain information from her surgeon as well as colleagues who had gone back to nursing, and she offered advice to women preparing for a new hip.

"The surgeon was quite helpful, and I was fortunate to be going to the private hospital that I chose because a lot of hip replacements were done there, and a couple of my friends from my nursing days had gone back to nursing and were working there. So I did get a bit of information from them about different aspects of the hospital and how you progressed. In our day we used to prepare patients for the operation, shave them with lots of soapy water and sharp razors. One nurse was telling me these horrific stories that they don't use soap and water any more. They just use dry shaving! I thought, Oh, heavens. Anyway she said, 'If you want my advice, go to one of those places where you have a full leg wax and bikini line and you'll be right.' So the day before I was going in, I went to the little beauty parlour nearby. At the hospital when the young nurse came in, I said, 'Look, I've had a full leg wax and bikini line.' She said, 'Oh, that's fine.' I recommend that."

Betty went to the hospital a week before the operation. There was no formal pre-admission clinic. At the time, her medical history was taken, she was advised to cease taking aspirin, and she signed an authority for the operation to be performed.

My experience and that of others strongly recommends attending the pre-admission clinic because it will show and tell you personally what you can expect from the hospital and help to allay your anxiety about the operation and hospital life.

Amusement while recovering

I gave little thought to the question of amusing myself while recovering until the last minute. I did not think that I would be reading much. I took in a small radio cassette tape recorder, and some music and books on tape. Mario felt much the same.

"I saw it as a time away from home. I'd be in bed for most of the time, and thought about music and books. I prepared myself for a lot of time without activity."

Ernst knew the exact date of his operation and recovery months before. He planned the operation to be after the national sporting championships in which he would be active, and his recovery would be during the Olympic Games, which he could watch on TV.

Like me, Helen found it most necessary to have some music.

"I had a friend's portable CD player. Sometimes you want to be by yourself, and you don't want to be available to be talked at. That was my private time with the music, and it was really good. Everyone respected it, too."

In most hospitals each bed has its own television set and radio. For active entertainment you might need your knitting, sewing bag, crossword dictionary, list of phone numbers, a writing pad, cards, envelopes, and stamps to catch up on correspondence. A tin of your own candies or sweets might be a treat to look forward to.

Your attitude to amusement and entertainment will change in a few days after the operation, and you will probably get bored, as many patients do, and then begin to ask your friends to bring you things you might not have thought about until then.

Feelings about and attitudes to the hip operation

How do you manage anxiety about being in hospital and having the operation?

Feeling anxious about the operation and recovery is normal. The environment and the people are unfamiliar, and hospitals are mainly known as places of emergencies, danger, panic, and medical heroics. You stay in hospital with strangers who are working for your recovery in an organisation that is a mystery, where there is great pressure on staff to be considerate and efficient in a culture of high tension over matters of life and death. So you will feel oddly anxious while others go coolly about their daily work.

Nurses are bound to care for you in a patient, tolerant, relaxed manner. You will be in pain, not feeling at all well, suffering from being dependent, and will easily see others as infantilising you. Feelings of irritation might grow, hackles begin to rise, tempers flare, and childish behaviour replaces the common sense of adulthood. Nurses, physiotherapists, and other medical staff often see this sort of behaviour in patients. Most medical staff handle signs of anxiety very well; they listen attentively and genuinely, don't argue or judge you, and hear what you say, what you do not say, and what you can't say without a little help. Nurses know you are feeling sick, nauseous, worrying about whether you can urinate or empty your bowels. Their nursing has taught them much on how sensitive you are about toileting, eating, not sleeping, vomiting, feeling wretched for no reason, being unclean, smelly, and looking unkempt and awful.

To manage your natural responses to illness, nurses try to find a productive way to work with you. You will notice nurses present a catalogue of unflappable, pleasant, caring, helpful characteristics. They appear to want you to feel better, get better, and leave the hospital and their care in good spirits. Outside the ward, during their coffee break, you can be sure that they will let off steam, joke, complain and issue warnings and vent their anger with amazing stories about miserable, thoughtless, demanding patients like you or the person in the next bed. In short, nurses are like all caring professionals; they know their job and have their own professional ways of coping with its problems.

What can you do to make their work meet your needs? Becoming a patient in a hospital is a like having a job. Work is given to you, real work, and expectations are held about your performance. At the same time you are focused on your work by the social life that surrounds you.

In the beginning your work as a patient is governed by the expectation that for a time you should be as dependent as a child is on its parents. This time is difficult for most adults. But if you accept this child-like dependence consciously for two or three days, your natural anxiety will diminish. If you refuse this child-like dependency, and fight to be in charge of the hospital and its staff, artificial or neurotic anxiety will probably emerge, and you will behave childishly. Most adults — and nurses are adults — find childishness in adults quite irritating and embarrassing, and that it makes the work of nursing ever more difficult. And nurses avoid patients who are noisy and complaining, who storm at authorities, demand everything at once, elaborate on stories of felt injustice, blame others excessively, and moralise with outrage. The work of a dependent adult in a childlike relationship can be performed effectively if you consciously relax and follow the gentle advice of nurses and physiotherapists on how to use your body as they suggest.

Terri expressed very well the emotionality of being a patient, and the way she used to dissociate the surgery from her self, until reality entered when her autologous blood donation became necessary.

> "I just wanted to be feeling as light and comfortable in myself. Whenever I get stressed and upset, I lose my appetite. That's how I cope with things. To deal emotionally with going into hospital when I know I'm having surgery, I say, 'I'm having a surgery and that's over there. I'm having a hip replacement. It's over there.' It wasn't until two weeks before the operation, when I had to start donating my blood, that it became a reality, and I started grieving, getting upset, getting tense, being horrible to live with, crying. As much as I needed surgery, I still had that emotional side to deal with."

I was emotional but in a different way. The weekend was coming up, and dear friends suggested staying the weekend with them at their beach house. We enjoyed the company, talk, and wine, had a few walks, and went on a picnic. I read and tried to occupy myself with matters unrelated to the operation. But the anxiety did not go away. It became manageable in small ways. Before we left to return to the city I sat for a photograph in a chair that I was greatly attracted to. Weeks later I saw the photograph with my face carrying a grave tribute to pain and anxiety.

In hospital all I had to do was remind myself that if I did not have the operation life would be intolerable, pain would be unbearable, and before long I would not be able to walk. My rationalised way of looking at the problem was to feel that I had no choice but surgery. And my surgeon was the best.

Mario believed little could be done, too. As he said:

> "There's obviously an inevitability about the whole thing. It has to be done."

Fred was anxious, too. Forty years earlier, as a young psychologist working in hospitals, he had watched operations firsthand and readily recalled the ineptness of surgeons, their clumsiness, and their lack of concern for the outcome of errors in operating procedures. Even so, after twenty years of pain he felt he had no choice. Doug was anxious and simply admitted that he was a coward for the few days that it was necessary to be one.

Bernard managed the anxiety with what he had learned from

the pre-admission clinic and advice from a neighbour and from his brother. Terri was as emotional as anyone could be, and let those close to her know it.

"I mean, it was an emotional thing. Sure, it's easy just to let them take the blood. But emotionally, having to face the surgery is hard. I remember I had a fight with my husband. He was supposed to take me down the first time. We had this fight, and I went by myself. I was miserable. I was so upset. I mean, it was because of having to have this surgery. I have times where I think, 'I'm sick of this disease. I've had enough.' I didn't want to have this operation. I didn't want to go through it. I just wanted the result."

On the other hand, Tess had been well prepared for her operation a thousand times because she had served as a theatre nurse all her professional life.

"I was feeling fine. Having seen a lot of surgery, it didn't bother me at all. I'm all for it. If anything's wrong, have it cut out. A lot of people aren't. But I felt, 'Oh yes. I'll have it done. I didn't mind it at all.' I didn't have any time to worry. I just came home and prepared a bag. I asked the surgeon, 'Am I going to have a spinal?' He said, 'In a way it's up to you. Discuss it with the anaesthetist. I'd prefer a general.' So I had a general."

4

Hospital life before the operation

Most people are admitted to hospital for their operation around the middle of the day. You may take with you a friend or relative who is expected to leave in the evening. After going to the front desk and being admitted as a patient, you sign documents and then go to the ward with a nurse. You learn where your bed is, and you are helped to settle in. Time passes, you are fed, and in the evening your anaesthetist calls to discuss how you will sleep during the operation.

Next day, the nursing staff prepare you for the operation, shave and clean you, ensure that you do not eat or drink too much — if indeed you are allowed anything — and help you into a special gown and a cap for your hair, and maybe some special underwear.

You may not take your usual medications; maybe your blood pressure will be taken and your blood tested. You might be X-rayed again. About a hour before the operation your receive a calming injection, and slowly you begin to drift into unconsciousness, more or less. Although people are talking to you and asking questions, the sense of what is being said is elusive, and the world seems a little hazy.

The nurse and others wheel you on your bed to the operating theatre where, after a little banter, your anaesthetist gives you an injection. And that's it. You wake up and it's over.

Arriving at the hospital

I was taken to the hospital at 2 p.m. on a Sunday and was to be operated on early the following day. Nervously I approached the reception desk and said who I was. I was told to wait in the lounge area across the foyer. I watched a bent old woman being helped to the elevator. I imagined I was just as old, and wondered why we bothered at our age.

A young nurse took me and my companion up two floors in a spacious elevator to the ward and showed me my room. I discovered equipment for two beds, not one as I had expected. I felt most ambivalent about the idea of being in a room with another person. Expecting that if you ask for single accommodation in a private hospital you get it, my helper went into action. The nurse in charge at her station nearby said that no private room was vacant and that when one did become available I would be put into it; meanwhile I could be assured that on this floor, in this ward, there lived one big, happy community. Very courteously and firmly the nurse put us in our place. Very quickly I learned that I was not in control; I was dependent on others. Accepting these two conditions was my first task.

When Doug booked into the hospital he felt angry. He had top insurance cover, had waited almost a year to qualify for it, and assumed that he would be put in a single, private room.

> "I found out the paperwork hadn't gone through as it should have. Where the problem came was when they assigned me to a bed in a six-bed ward. And here I'm going to what was supposed to be a private hospital. I'd put my money in to come to a private room. So I got pretty upset about that. They made assurances to me that as soon as a private or semi-private ward was vacant they would transfer me."

Doug did not forget his discontent easily. After the operation he suffered serious complications, and certainly did not appreciate having five other patients in the room sharing his misery.

> "I was having a bit of difficulty shortly after the operation. When I was sick, having people around me, not just people attending me but all these other people, concerned me. And it was rammed home at that particular moment that if I'd had the room I wanted, I wouldn't be so worried about it."

Charles had no trouble at all. He was on the second highest level of the health insurance table, and when he was admitted to the hospital he got a private room. Nell felt that she did so by good luck.

"I stipulated to a few people that I didn't want visitors. I'm like a cat. If I'm not well I prefer to be alone. And that worked very well. I had a private room. I was lucky right from the beginning. Even if you've got top cover you don't always get that."

On the other hand, Bernard had a surgeon who preferred his patients in a private room, but the hospital was so busy that he was put in a three-bed ward and stayed there all the time. He would have preferred a private room for a few days, but since everyone else with him was sick he supposed it would be all right.

Mario was untroubled by the hospital's decision. Five years earlier he had gone to a private hospital where he shared a room, and today nothing stands out that was inappropriate at that time.

"I went with the flow. What happened seemed appropriate."

But Terri, like Doug, was terribly upset by her treatment at the time of admission, although she had been to hospital for her illness before.

"I always want to have a private room. When I checked in they took me to a room I thought was my room. It wasn't in the orthopaedic ward. I unpacked my bag and started settling in. Then we moved to another room before surgery, and even that wasn't the one I was staying in. Three days after the operation they moved me to another one. Of course by then, you're totally immobile; you can't move your things yourself. I wish they had found my room, let me get settled, grounded, and know where I was going to be. I understand their point of view if they haven't got the room available at that time."

The day Betty had her operation she was taken to the hospital by a friend. The room seemed not to matter; she was grateful to get in anywhere because she needed to have the operation so badly.

It is clear that private health insurance does not entitle you to a private single room in a private hospital. Once you are admitted to hospital your accommodation is in the hands of the hospital administration and nurses. They might offer single accommodation, but they can never guarantee it.

Settling in

The world around me began to shrink and concentrate itself on my body. I was advised that I should get into my night clothes and wait for dinner. A uniformed waitress came to offer me a glass of sherry. Sipping it slowly, I thought this was not a bad hotel. Later came a delicious dinner. My friend returned in time to watch television. I was then put to bed and learned that the following day at 2 p.m. I was to have the operation and would not be eating for hours beforehand. Settling in seemed effortless.

Doug did not settle in well at first. He was put into the worst bed in the ward, an old-style one.

> "The newer beds have a winding handle, so they can wind you up or wind you down. Being in an older bed caused a little bit of trouble. They did change my bed to the wind-up one. It was so much easier to use."

Helen, a strict vegetarian who was doing her university research into meat culture in the hospital, had a deep interest in controlling her diet. Immediately she was in conflict with the hospital's catering authorities.

> "As an experiment this time I went into this private hospital as a **vegan**, just to see what they would do. I felt they starved me, stuffed up my diet, and made me really thin and pasty. So I was continually talking to the kitchen about their inability to feed me properly."

Preparing you for the operation

Showering and shaving

Early on the day of the operation a nurse came to shave me. Forty years earlier I had had an operation on my spine; then a male barber had come to shave every hair from my body from the waist down to my knees with a cut-throat razor! Here stood this young woman, apparently planning to do the same with an electric razor. She showed me on her own body where she would be shaving me. She shaved me in a decorous manner, and at no time did I feel embarrassed.

Next came the shower. She said I had to be as free of germs as possible. She gave me a tube of clear, green fluid and advised me that every part of my body needing washing. An hour before the operation I had to have another shower and was instructed to dress in a long white gown that tied at the back.

Mario could not recall the shave, but did remember washing.

"I had a shower with a special sort of stuff all over me. I didn't realise that was going to happen. I certainly didn't know before that."

A quite different technique was used on Bernard.

"To shave that part of my hip they just rubbed cream on it. They rubbed cream right to my feet, right down the whole lot. Then they just sponged it off. For the few spots left, the nurse just got the razor and gave it a bit of a flick. That morning I got up, and I went and had a shower with antiseptic yellowy-green stuff."

Betty remembered:

"You had to be shaved and all that. There was a male nurse, very attentive. Before the operation took place I had showers with white soap. It was mainly an antiseptic, and we had to shower ourselves."

In the belief that she would be subject to a dry shave Wendy had gone to a beauty parlour a day before going to the hospital and had herself shaved to the bikini line.

Blood testing

The moment I was given a bed at the hospital, my blood pressure was measured, and blood samples were taken regularly by nurses from the pathology clinic at the hospital. Blood pressure assessment seemed to be something nurses did every few hours. Bernard also recalled nurses regularly taking blood tests.

Your consent to be a patient

Your surgeon needs legal permission to operate on you, so at some time before the operation you will be expected to sign a consent form. I signed such a form, and to this day I can say honestly that I did not understand it. Later I learned that, among other things, the form gave the surgeon my informed consent — that is, I knew what the operation was for and wanted to have it — to do what he thought best if the unexpected occurred while I was being operated on.

I trusted the surgeon fully to do the best he could no matter what; and I knew at the time, because he had told me, that I was risking infection, dislocation, and a blood clot. I was prepared to accept all of those risks. I did not know that by signing the form I was allowing the surgeon to do what he thought fit in a emergency without seeking the permission of my next of kin, who at the time was aged 90, sprightly, and sound asleep in his bed a hundred kilometres (60 miles) away.

Although I believe I read the consent form thoroughly, I certainly did not understand it fully. Why? It was in legal language and difficult to follow; I was feeling very anxious and not keen to decode legalisms; and I was sleepy because of drugs given to prepare me for the operation. At the time I believe I was not anxious about the content of the form. I was anxious to get a new hip. If the consent form had been available at the time of the pre-admission clinic, enquiries into its meaning and significance could have been taken up then.

Only a lawyer can tell you precisely what the consent form says and means. For practical purposes it says that you understand as well as a non-specialist can what is to be done with your body, why it is about to be done, and that you agree to having it done. Also, if a medical crisis occurs during the preparation, operation, and recovery, you agree that the surgeon and those helping the surgeon should act immediately in your vital interests according to their best judgment at the time. In everyday terms this means you know you are going to have the hip operation, you trust the surgeon you have chosen, and you believe your surgeon will be doing their best to make you better. If you feel anxious about whatever you think the form says, ask questions until you no longer feel anxious.

Betty too had to sign an authority, not just before the operation but a week earlier.

"I think I had to give them authority to do it. And give them my next of kin. That would've been the week before."

Nell did the same and enjoyed the amusing thought that she would not be able to blame anyone even if the worst happened.

"I had to sign a whole lot of things to say that I wouldn't hold them responsible if I dropped dead, I suppose. That was at the desk before I went to my room."

Charles, a lawyer, was much amused by having to sign a form relating to an experiment on anticoagulant drugs for which he was asked to be a subject shortly before the operation. The researchers, including his surgeon and other colleagues, had to follow the nation's ethical guidelines for medical researchers who used human subjects. The research investigated the relative efficacy of two drugs, **Clexane** and **warfarin**, used to prevent blood clots.

"Clexane was used to prevent blood clotting in lieu of warfarin. It's a new venture, they were looking for guinea pigs, and I agreed to do it. They approached me on the night before the operation. Would I be in this? So I was in a fairly accommodating mood at that stage. I had to sign the usual consent. I was very careful about consent forms. My legal training led to my putting in some conditions, crossing out some clauses. They can't contract themselves out of negligence, anyway. I think I wrote that somewhere. One of them wasn't very impressed by what I wrote. They came along with another form when I was lying on the trolley in the room waiting to go into the theatre, wanting me to sign. I said, 'I'm damned if I'm going to sign anything now at this stage.' "

Of course if you are asked to sign the form shortly before the operation as Charles and I were, when you are far from clear-headed, you would probably be within your rights not to sign. But would the surgeon be willing to operate if you refuse to sign?

The anaesthetist's visit

I was most anxious about the anaesthetic. Forty years earlier I had come out of a general anaesthetic feeling very unwell and had no reason to think things would be different this time. I had heard that now there are two kinds of anaesthetic. The first was not much different from what I had experienced so long ago. It would close down my body fully. The other kind of anaesthetic was more localised, more specific to that part of the body being operated on: an **epidural**. A friend had told me that with an epidural he had heard voices during his operation! That really worried me. I did not want to hear anything. I felt anxious and was ignorant, and said nothing to anybody. Late in the evening on the day before the operation the anaesthetist appeared and introduced himself. I asked what kind of anaesthetic was planned. He said it would be an epidural. I wondered: would it put me to sleep entirely? I said I would be very pleased to have a general anaesthetic.

I felt that the anaesthetist could see I was puzzled and anxious. He assured me that the appropriate anaesthetic was an epidural, and that it had the advantage of a less distressing recovery than the general anaesthetic. I felt anxious because I imagined that I would be awake during the operation and could hear what was happening to me, although I would not feel any pain. I said nothing of this to the anaesthetist. Perhaps he sensed my concern. He told me that an epidural would be used, that it involved an injection somewhere in my back, close to the spine, and that I would not be aware of anything at all. Then he told me that, for about an hour before the operation, I would be lightly drugged and feeling quite relaxed. I believed him, trusted him, and felt much better.

The anaesthetic was a major issue for Sonomi and raised a problem that gave her more concern than any other aspect of her hip replacement. Sonomi was determined that she would not have an epidural anaesthetic. Years ago, experiences in her home country, the USA, informed her that the epidural block, commonly used in childbirth, had serious side effects that she believed were far too hazardous to her health and welfare. She told her story to the nurses at the pre-admission clinic, and they recommended strongly that she take up the question with her anaesthetist. She wanted to discuss the matter with her anaesthetist in private, yet when she approached him on the eve of her operation, he was not prepared to talk with her in private. She was distressed and angered by this. In time he was able to find a place nearby for a private discussion and, after hearing what she had to say, agreed on a general anaesthetic.

Charles's anaesthetist talked with him the night before the operation.

"I knew about the pre-med injections because I had had one before. I had a sporting injury in the leg, so I knew what to expect. Epidural. I think he said that."

Mario was not interested in the anaesthetic and did not recall any options being given or any trauma associated with it. Bernard was disabused of a popular fear about anaesthetics and, with help from others, became well informed about its consequences. His brother had had an epidural and told Bernard that he had been awake. So Bernard, like Sonomi, was keen to have a general anaesthetic.

"I would've preferred to be done the old way with chloroform. General anaesthetic. And I thought, 'Well, they prefer to do it with the other way, with a spinal.' I thought, 'I'm going to be laying there listening to the saws cutting through bone.' The anaesthetist said, 'You'll doze off. You won't know a thing about being in the theatre.' "

Wendy, in spite of her experience as a nurse, was anxious about the anaesthetic, and wondered what new developments had occurred since she had left work to be a full-time mother. When she was nursing, spinal anaesthetics were not used.

"The anaesthetist came in the night before. He said, 'You're fine. The only thing we have to decide now is whether you have a general or a spinal.' I said, 'I don't want a spinal. I don't want to be awake for this. I want to be right out to it.' I thought that with a spinal your brain would be awake. He said, 'Look, you'll have a pre-med and you'll be pretty dopey. You won't know much about it. You're better off with that than a general. It's up to you, but that's what I would recommend.' I said, 'Well, as long as you say that I'll be pretty dopey.' "

Terri described her close relationship with her anaesthetist when she explained what was going to happen to her.

"The anaesthetist was great. She came on three different occasions after the surgery to see how I was going. I've never had that before. She went through the options with me, and we decided on an epidural block. We decided on the epidural block because it could be left in for two days afterwards, for two pain-free days. I don't tolerate **pethidine** or **morphine** very well. I just start throwing up. And so that was the best option. Well, they do a light general anaesthetic anyway, because they don't want you awake during the operation. But all I remember is going down to the room."

Helen was not informed about the anaesthetic.

"I was cared for, but I was never informed. What sort of anaesthetic? I wouldn't have a clue. There was no discussion. He came to see me the night before, but he was only there for five seconds. It's only when the bill comes that you know who the anaesthetist was. Always, always, there's been very, very little information."

These experiences reinforce the recommendation that if you do not understand what will be happening to you, simply ask. If you do not get the information you want, demand it. If you feel reassured and secure about the events that are about to take place, your recovery will probably be far less stressful and more rapid, and both you and the medical staff will benefit.

A year later I spoke with an anaesthetist about the experiences of the patient and the popular meanings attaching to technical terms like *epidural*, *spinal*, *epidural block*, *general anaesthetic*, and so forth. We discussed the question of being conscious and unconscious, awake or asleep, dopey and alert, remembering and forgetting. One reason for the anxiety you naturally feel about an operation centres on the question of whether you will feel, sense or know anything or in any way have a normal grasp of your own presence at the operation. Be assured that you will not, no matter what technical term is attached to the anaesthetic. That is the avowed aim of the anaesthetist.

The work of the anaesthetist is curious in two ways: on one hand, the task is to ensure that the patient is out to it, and on the other hand, that your body functions as normally as possible. The anaesthetist is greatly helped in this work if you are a non-smoker, not overweight, as physically fit as possible, and as free of anxiety as possible. If you are highly anxious, make sure the anaesthetist knows, for only then can he or she help you to be a competent patient.

Pre-operative activities

Timing of the operation

On the morning of the operation I was told that there had been delays and that I would have to be put into a queue and wait until the evening. This allowed me to have a hot drink and a biscuit or cookie, but nothing more. I was not interested in eating. Friends sat with me during the day, and about five o'clock the action began.

Doug was delayed, too. His operation was to be done in the morning, but, for reasons not made clear to him, it was done in the evening. On the other hand, Mario and Bernard were done quite swiftly after their admission to the hospital. Wendy went to some trouble to ensure that she was not kept waiting. She registered at the private hospital, which her surgeon used regularly, on the day before the operation, and, because the hospital was small and she knew the nursing staff, she asked if she could be first cab off the rank next day. Sonomi was also first cab off the rank, but she had had no influence with the hospital at all.

This illustrates the point that, once you are in hospital, the events that lead up to the operation are well outside your control, unless you have some special relationship with the hospital staff. It is probably best to do as Mario did and go with the flow.

Feeling drugged and woozy

About an hour before the operation I was injected with some drug, quickly relaxed, and felt very comfortable. Gradually I gained the impression that my concentration was fading and that I was not speaking as crisply as I usually did. People began smiling at me. It was getting close to the time for the operation. People said 'Goodbye' and wished me luck. I felt in high spirits as a group of white uniforms wheeled me and my bed into an elevator and then to the operating theatre.

Doug found the drug was not effective as he had been led to believe.

> "I had no reaction whatsoever. I was waiting for it, still as anxious as ever, and nothing seemed to happen. So I told them. The anaesthetist said it was OK."

To make things worse, there seemed to Doug to be some misunderstanding about why he was having an operation. It is common practice for you to be asked your name when you arrive at the theatre, which operation you think you are having, what side of your body is involved, and for apparently light-hearted talk to prevail. As Doug said:

> "There were jokes. 'I believe it's the right testicle we're removing.' And: 'It's the one on the left side, isn't it?' And I keep telling them that it's the right side."

Charles was treated quite differently before the operation and given a clear responsibility to prepare for the operation himself.

> "I walked the streets to get my circulation going, which they advised me to do until an hour before, and then I put on my pyjamas and let the medical staff get on with it. I just mentally accepted it. By the time I got into the operating area, I was pretty dopey and groggy."

In the operating theatre

I felt fine. I had a desultory conversation with the anaesthetist. He suggested that I roll on to my left side while he injected something into my back. I felt quite happy with that, but sensed he had some problem. I could feel light pricking around the middle of my spine, and heard him saying to me quite clearly that he was finding it hard to settle on a place to inject me. I was quite unconcerned and imagined he would find somewhere to put it.

Doug remembered that in the operating theatre:

> "... they virtually folded me up into a foetal position, and they said, 'This won't be uncomfortable.' I didn't feel it go in, but my left leg straightened. Must have been a nerve they hit. It was a strange sensation to have that happen without my doing it. I was out completely. Didn't hear anything."

Bernard was tested for the effect of the anaesthetic.

> "They just wheeled me, bed and all, into the theatre, put the needle in, and asked, 'Can you lift your feet?' I tried to lift my feet but I couldn't."

Terri smiled as she recalled those few moments before the anaesthetic took hold.

> "My nicest time was pre-operative when I was with my anaesthetist. She said, 'Oh, you're so chatty', and I know I was just talking, talking, talking. We were having a really nice, interesting conversation, and I do remember her telling me to curl up to get the needle in. I remember she couldn't find where she wanted to do things, and she said, 'I'll do that when you're

under.' What I find is sort of annoying is that I know I was awake for a lot more of the time, but I can't remember it."

Betty could remember some of the theatre banter just before she went under, and Wendy had hazy recollections of events before the operation.

"People talking and a bit of noise, but I had no sense of time. I had the pre-med half an hour before I went down, and they might have given me something during it, another little booster, I don't know. But certainly I have no recollection of being aware of what was going on. You put your faith in them."

The operation itself

Most patients recall little about the operation and seem to prefer it that way. The last thing they remember is the drowsiness after being given an injection to help them relax. The drug also dries out the lungs a little and makes breathing easy when you sleep.

Only those in the operating theatre can describe fully the details of the operation. My surgeon told people that my old hip was pretty bad, nothing more. Interested readers can see the details of the operation in an atlas of hip replacement, or on a film in a medical library, or in a museum among the medical exhibits.

What follows is a non-technical summary of the major events during a hip replacement operation.

If you have an epidural anaesthetic a needle goes into an area beside your spine, so that anaesthetic surrounds the spinal cord and numbs you from the waist down. You are also given a sedative to keep you unconscious. If you have a general anaesthetic your body is closed down; you are unconscious and feel nothing.

Once you are asleep, you are usually given a drug to paralyse your muscles so that the anaesthetist can control your breathing with a tube that goes down your throat. Your lungs are ventilated well, the chances of lung infections are reduced, and with your muscles paralysed your surgeon can manipulate your hip easily.

In a deep sleep you are lifted on to the narrow operating table and placed in a position for the surgeon to begin work. Half a dozen trained staff are there to help in the surgical part of the operation, which will last perhaps eighty to ninety minutes. The area around the cut is washed with an antiseptic, dried, and covered with a drape. An incision is made, and bleeding is stopped artificially as the cut is deepened. The hip is dislocated. The knobby head of the femur is sawn off at the neck and taken aside by the theatre nurse to be used later if necessary. The acetabulum — the socket — is now obvious, and, using an instrument like a cheese cutter, the surgeon reams the socket to the desired shape, about 50–56 mm across. Men have a larger pelvis than women. If the acetabulum is to have a cemented layer on it, small holes are drilled in the **reamed** surface to help bond the new hip to the old bone. Meanwhile the theatre nurse prepares the cement, and the surgeon puts it into the cleaned socket under pressure. As the cement begins to harden, the surgeon pushes in the plastic cup and waits for the cement to set. If no cement is used, a metal backing for the acetabulum is hammered into the socket and might be fixed with small screws. The plastic cup is clicked into the metal backing.

Next the femur is prepared. A cylindrical reamer makes a central channel down the inside of the femur through the marrow. If cement is used, a plug is put into the femur to prevent the cement from vanishing from the end of the bone when the time comes to put it in from the top. The femur is washed, dried, and filled with cement, and the metal stem of the prosthesis is pushed well into the femur and held steady until the cement sets. If it is a cementless procedure, the prothesis stem is fitted snugly into the carefully reamed femur.

Finally, the ball of the ball and socket is fitted to the stem of the femoral segment, and the socket and ball are pressed together into a new hip joint. Adjustments are made to ensure that your legs are about the same length; antibiotics might be used to lower the chances of infection; tests are done to see that the likelihood of dislocation is reduced and that the hip is secure and stable. The wound is closed, and often drains are inserted to remove oozing blood. Finally, the operated leg is strapped at the ankles to a triangular abduction pillow to ensure that the hip is stable at the time you wake in a high-dependency or recovery room. In such a room emergency equipment is available to cope with any complications that might occur, e.g. difficulties of breathing and swallowing.

If the operation is uneventful, the whole procedure, from leaving the ward to returning to it, takes between one and two hours. With the preparation and recovery time included, you will be unavailable for between six and eight hours.

Many precautions are taken to ensure that your recovery is routine. Because blood can pool in your legs during the operation, white thromboembolic deterrent (TED) stockings, also known as deep vein thrombosis (DVT) stockings, are put on your legs. So you wake up with white stockinged legs if that is your surgeon's practice. Also, if you need it, you will have a blood transfusion, injections of antibiotics to reduce infection, and blood thinning injections or tablets to make sure that blood clots do not occur.

In the recovery room you will find yourself wearing a light, clear oxygen mask. There will be a drip in your arm for the painkiller and other necessary fluids, drains coming from your wound, and, if necessary, a **catheter** taking away your urine. If you recover routinely, in a few hours you will be taken back to your ward. You might feel bright and cheerful; you might feel tired and sick, with a headache.

In your new hip is the prosthesis, a stem and ball of cobalt or titanium-based alloys, and a special bone cement like that used by dentists to hold things together, if necessary. In the socket is a variety of tough plastic, ultra high molecular weight polyethylene. These substances are all compatible with the tissues and bone of the human body.

Waking up

Bright sun was shining, and I felt warm, soft, and comfortable. I glimpsed people sitting to my right and smiling. I asked, 'What's the time?' 10.30 a.m. 'Well, that was quick, wasn't it?' I said, feeling pleased and happy. When I saw the tray in front of me, I tore away the clear plastic mask over my mouth and nose, and lashed into the coffee and cornflakes. A smiling nurse materialised to tell me that I would stay a while in this recovery room with a line of operated people. I craned to see in the bed directly opposite that elderly woman I had seen tottering in the foyer two days ago. She had had her operation before me. What happened to her? Two new knees at the age of 90! I was most impressed.

Doug was feeling quite bright when he woke up at half past eight in the morning.

"I spoke with my wife on the phone. I didn't have any pain. I was hooked up to the epidural still dripping into me, and a catheter had been put in to save me going to the toilet. Later they gave me something to eat."

Mario quickly phoned his wife, too.

"I was in bed in the ward. And I fairly quickly made a phone call, I think, in a groggy state, trying to remember the phone number and then trying to reach the phone. I think I spoke to my wife to let her know I was all right. She told me to get off the phone. I think she was surprised that I did ring."

Charles was operated on about one o'clock in the afternoon.

"I didn't wake up till about half past five or six. I think just the nurse was there when I woke up in the room. That was my first impression. I presume I did go to a recovery room, but I didn't wake up there. But I started to get better. It was sporadic, really. I'd have a bit to eat, and then start again."

Terri woke in the recovery room.

"There was a mask over my face and things coming out all directions. And, boy, did I need to have a pee. Pethidine doesn't do much for my pain. It makes me drowsy. I didn't get a trip with it. I had the epidural in still, and they can position it so it works down the side that you've been operated on. So my left leg was pretty numb, and I could use my other leg. That was great. Whenever I had to go to the loo, I had to push to go. I didn't expect that. I really had to concentrate."

Nell did not see her anaesthetist in the morning before the operation because she was unconscious before she went down to the operating theatre.

"Before I got to the theatre they gave me some sort of tablet, and it made me more than woozy. It knocked me right out. Next thing I knew they were calling me to wake up. I said, 'Oh, is it time to go down?' And they said, 'No. You're back already.'"

Like Mario and Charles, Bernard woke up in the ward, not the recovery room.

"Nobody else was there, not at that stage. I was pretty well bombed out, sort of half awake, and I thought, 'Oh yes, I'm back in the room.' I had a window bed looking out at pine trees outside. I rang the wife on the phone, and she said, 'Oh, you're drunk.' "

And, like Bernard, Ernst made an unusual phone call to his wife.

"I made a strange phone call to my wife. The operation finished about 8.30 p.m., and at 11.30 or 12 o'clock that night I persuaded the nurse in the intensive care that I was fine. Apparently I seemed lucid. I have no memory of it at all. I rang my wife and made a very strange phone call about religious things and so on, which is not me at all."

$$\left(5\right)$$

Recovery — the first few days

You should expect to be in hospital for about ten days, cared for by nurses and physiotherapists. As you recover, you might see an occupational therapist and social workers, who will help you with your immediate future when you leave the hospital. Although ten days in hospital seems to be the usual period, Ernst was there for only five and Nell stayed for fifteen days.

Immediately after the operation, your visitors will find you feeling weary, if not completely shocked, groggy, nauseous, and perhaps complaining of a headache. Nevertheless, some people come out of the anaesthetic feeling quite well and cheerful. There will be an intravenous **drip** in your wrist or thereabouts, and tubes will be draining excess fluid from your wound into bottles out of sight below the bed.

On waking up you will be free of hip pain because the anaesthetist will have given you drugs to kill pain in the wound and to prevent you from vomiting. A few hospitals have a system called PCA (**patient–controlled analgesia**), whereby the patient controls the analgesic under final control by the staff. If you find you are a PCA patient, be assured that you cannot overdose yourself, because the dosage is limited to the amount determined earlier by your doctors.

For a day after the operation you can expect nurses to give you close care and attention that is aimed at alleviating pain, preventing **thrombosis**, and managing feelings of nausea. Your physiotherapist will appear and encourage you to move your new hip a little and see whether you can begin to regain confidence in wiggling your leg. Nurses will continue to hover. They will take blood tests

intravenous line

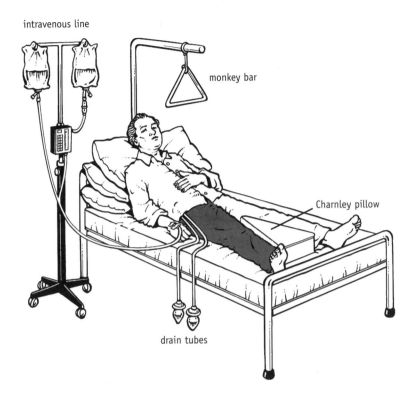

monkey bar

Charnley pillow

drain tubes

Figure 5: In bed in the ward soon after the operation.

to measure your haemoglobin and to see whether you need more blood for any reason.

Only three things can go wrong: dislocation; infection; and deep vein thrombosis. These possible complications are discussed later in the chapter.

My informants' interest in the first two days after the operation centred on sleeping, pain relief, discomfort in bed, and what they thought were the effects of the anaesthetic.

Sleep and sleeping problems

In the first few hours after the operation I slipped in and out of sleep, hovering on the border of consciousness. I was interrupted by the arrival of flowers and dreams of great comfort and astounding interest, all of which have been forgotten. They came and went, and, just like the best of one's friends, stayed a while, drifted out, then came back, always welcome. In one dream I got out of bed, strode to the elevator, down to the foyer, across the parking lot, got into my car, and started it. I had difficulty changing gears. I woke trying to engage the clutch with my left foot and found someone had strapped a triangular cushion to it! I mentioned this to a nurse. She smiled and mumbled, 'Pethidine.' I said I wanted more. She smiled. 'We'll see.' A few days later the drip into my left wrist was removed, and I was given tablets for the discomfort of the wound. That ended the delightful dreaming.

While I found sleeping easy and enjoyable, Charles and Nell found it a scary, lasting problem. Nell daydreamed too but did not enjoy it.

> "I don't know what anaesthetic they used. But I think on the second day or second night, I was on pethidine, and that's awful. I saw spiders. I can see them now. I'll never forget them."

Charles was harassed by dreadful images.

> "I had all the creepy-crawlies on the ceiling. Hallucinations. What upset me was having to sleep on my back, because I didn't sleep. With that pillow between my legs, I really didn't sleep more than an hour at a time, for about twelve weeks."

Sleeping on one's back is a common cause of sleep problems. Many people seem to have no way to prepare for it. I did not have an serious objection to lying on my back, except that, as time went by, a most irritating rash developed.

After the operation the first few days lying down were difficult for both Bernard and Terri but for different reasons. Bernard recalled the strictures of his surgeon regarding movement in bed and found the nurses just as adamant about what he could and could not do in bed.

> "I didn't sleep much at all while I was in hospital, really. I can't sleep on my back, and you're not allowed to sleep any other way. I've never slept on my back. I just dozed every now and then. The surgeon wouldn't allow me to have a sleeping tablet of any sort in case I went into a deep sleep and

rolled over, or did something silly. He does that with all his patients. I asked the nurses, 'Please, could I have a sleeper? I've been hours without sleep.' They said, 'Mr W — [the surgeon] won't be pleased.' They wouldn't give me anything."

Terri also found she could not sleep on her back, but she found a way to manage the discomfort associated with her resting.

"I slept on my back. I found it very uncomfortable. No turning over, but they did ask, 'Do you want to put the pillow up there, and we'll try and turn you?' I tried to vary my sleep by lying down, and then by sitting up with one pillow, then by sitting up with two pillows, and then I lay down again. That was my variation for sleep."

Pain, discomfort, and relief

A clear plastic tube, attached at the other end to a glass jar, was inserted into my left arm above my wrist and suspended high above my head on the right of the bed. Some time passed before I was aware of the tube. Fluid was dripping down the tube into my body. I believe it was to help me with dehydration — I am not sure — the fluid also contained a painkiller. Slowly the mixture dripped into my wrist and kept me in a sleepy, comfortable state.

Wendy was happy, too, with the efforts to relieve her pain.

"The continuous morphine was very good as far as pain relief. I had a continuous saline and morphine drip. And that was good."

By contrast, Nell had not expected so much pain after the operation.

"I was surprised at the pain afterwards. I wasn't expecting it. I went into it blithely, thinking, 'I'm going to get rid of this pain.' In the groin pain was all round, all round the back, the front, everywhere. I suppose it was fortunate that I didn't know it was going to be such a very painful process afterwards. But you get through these things."

Mario had injections that he believed might have relieved his pain but, at the same time, seemed intended to reduce the chances of infection.

"I think my first impression was that the pain had gone, closely followed by the spread-eagled position in the bed, that fixed position, with the pillow between my legs. The other realities were a sore back, perhaps from being in a fixed position, perhaps something from the operation. That was resolved by getting a special mattress overlay, which changed the bed from being totally flat to being ribbed. And the two other discomforts were the continual injections — I've never quite got used to them — in the stomach. I didn't like those injections because they stung a little bit. I don't know what it was. The injections were to avoid some sort of infection, an antibiotic, two or three times a day. That went on for a while. And there was a second discomfort, the drainage tube. The removal of that from the wound was fairly painful."

Ernst, who would leave hospital on the fifth day, was a remarkably fit man. He was married to a doctor, who cared for him at home. He had so little pain after the first operation that he was surprised to find the degree of pain increase markedly in the second operation. He was allowed to use patient–controlled analgesia to manage his pain.

"After the first operation, I had a little bit of superficial pain in the wound. I used a bit of **paracetamol** in hospital if I wanted to sleep. After the second operation, because of more swelling, I had more pain. I was using **Panadeine Forte** to sleep, and I think I got hooked on the codeine part of it. The second time I had a bit of pain because of bruising, and he hooked me up with a thing that I could use to give myself morphine, but I never used it because I had no pain. Not all anaesthetists are keen on it, I presume because the equipment is expensive. I think the hospital only had two or three of these set-ups, which could supply painkiller in patient-initiated amounts. There is a limit on it. I left hospital on day 5 each time, and the first time I went back to work after two and a half weeks."

Bernard had little pain and felt himself getting better as each day passed.

"I had three bottles hanging out of the hip, draining, and the morphine, or whatever. I got an injection in the stomach every night from the blood people. Not a lot of pain attached to it. For the first few days it's all inconvenience really, no great hassle about pain or anything. I knew I had a great gash in my leg, but I felt myself getting better every day."

For Doug, the pain of the operation and the wound were not as bad as the discomfort in bed and the nurse's attempts to move him.

> "Being turned over in bed was probably the most uncomfortable thing because you don't want to be moving around. That's the hardest part of it, I think. On your back for so many days."

Effects of the anaesthetic

People respond differently to anaesthetics. Some people have remarkable allergies to anaesthetics, others take a week or two to recover from them. I do not recall any effect on me that I can attribute to the anaesthetic itself apart from pleasant hallucinations. Years earlier I had had a operation and woke to several days of severe illness. I do not recall having told the anaesthetist that, but I might have done so when we talked about the epidural anaesthetic that he proposed using. As it turned out, he had to use a general anaesthetic, and my unhappy tales from forty years ago might have contributed to his decision to use pethidine. So I did not suffer at all. But Charles suffered greatly from the anaesthetic and felt that he was responsible.

> "The anaesthetic played up with me. I just got sick. Vomiting and things like that. Didn't eat for two or three days. It was probably my fault because, when they give you the form asking, 'Are you allergic to this and this?' I just said, 'No, no, no, no.' Because as far as I knew I wasn't. They think it was the morphine."

Morphine affected Wendy adversely too, but she was quickly given another painkiller.

> "I didn't react well to the morphine. I was allergic to it. I was very nauseated for several days afterwards. I really wasn't able to keep much down, and we got a physician eventually, and he put in a drip and put in some things that got me back on track. I was as good as gold. The hip was fine, but it was just this nausea."

Helen regarded morphine as the prime cause of her response to the anaesthetic three years earlier. She had been so sick that she was determined not to let it happen again.

"This time was very different from three years ago when I had the other side done. Then I was given a lot of morphine. I threw up continually for two weeks. I was not able to talk to anyone. I was just lying there, feeling like death warmed up. This time I told them not to give me morphine, and they didn't, and it was remarkable how different it was. I've never had much pain. Pethidine just didn't make me sick. I didn't get a buzz out of it as everyone says. I think they're a bit careless with the giving of morphine. While I was in hospital, one of the women next to me had her knee done, she was given morphine, and she almost died."

Terri was nauseated for a day or two and took charge of fluid consumption herself.

"I didn't eat that day. When I got back to the ward I was drinking, and I remember one nurse saying, 'Well, you really shouldn't be drinking as much as you are.' But I know myself what I can or can't do. I had just little sips of water. I didn't care for food at all the first day."

Terri had an epidural block, which involves leaving a small needle in the back for a day or so to manage pain. A problem arose when the needle was due to be removed. It would not come out, the anaesthetist was not available, and the nurses were anxious about making a mistake if they pulled it out too violently. This became a nightmare for Terri, because of what she imagined might be the outcome of the failure to get the epidural out of her back at the right time.

"My worst day after the surgery was the third day when the epidural was to come out in the morning, and the nurses said, 'Oh, look, it's not coming out.' I'm thinking, 'What the hell is going on here?' And they said, 'We're not going to pull it because we can get into trouble.' And I read between the lines, 'You don't want to be liable.' They said, 'We've got to get an anaesthetist.' And they couldn't get my anaesthetist. They had to find any anaesthetist. I was getting more upset by the minute, and it was in there until the middle of the afternoon before they got it out. And of course I was just about hysterical. 'Why isn't this coming out? Am I going to be left a cripple because this is in the wrong spot or something?' I was very fearful. They did locate an anaesthetist, and he came and he pushed me forward. I was told you don't go forward like that — and he pushed me forward! — and I thought, 'What are you doing to my joint if I'm not meant to do this movement?' The reason was that because I'm a young person, my muscles had closed in around the needle, whereas in older people, the muscles aren't as tight and don't constrict as easily. That explanation came later on."

Ernst had a problem with his anaesthetic that was kept from him until after the operation.

"I think I was very fortunate that I wasn't knocked around by the anaesthetic, and I recovered very quickly. I had a spinal the first time; the second time it was with a light general. Apparently the first time, when they gave me the sedative just before the spinal, I had a paradoxical reaction where they had to have three people to hold me down on the table. The anaesthetist came round a few days later, and he said, 'Are you all right?' I asked him why. He asked, 'No headaches?' 'No, I'm fighting fit.' He said, 'I had such trouble getting the lumbar puncture into the spine. Usually people have a headache after it. We had to get three people to hold you down. You were thrashing around.' I was unconscious, of course. Can't remember it at all."

Eating again

Food might interest you when you wake up because you will not have eaten for many hours. I was starving and ate a great breakfast. Others find they cannot eat for days. Light food and a sip of something might be best; the next day meals will offered to you regularly, unless you are feeling sick to the stomach.

I was thirsty and drank much water. My memory of this time is vague, but the food was excellent. People fussed around me and provided tea, coffee, and water. The physician noted that my stomach was becoming bloated because the fluid I was drinking was not getting through the usual channels. Without explanation I was put on a day-long diet of light, fluid-like food. I was given no gourmet food, only thin soup and jelly! I was furious. Where's the gourmet cooking? Politely I was told that 'Doctor' had 'put me on to fluids', and that was the way it was going to be until he changed his mind. He did so a day later when my waistline deflated. This move produced five litres of urine in one day.

Charles, Mario, and Bernard thought the food was good and

ate well. But before her surgery Terri had lost her appetite and some weight.

> "I did start eating the second day. I didn't enjoy the food. Towards the end I started to enjoy some meals, but it was a chore to eat the second day, and those early days."

Toilet achievements and embarrassments

There is a one in a hundred chance that you might have bowel troubles. Your bowels are close to your acetabulum, which will have taken quite a few heavy blows during the operation, and will take some time to recover from the shock. Nurses say that bowel trouble passes in a few days. But if it does not, and some infection emerges in your gastrointestinal tract, it is probably due to the antibiotics that have been used to prevent infection. The antibiotics tend to eliminate the usual bacteria that keep the intestines in normal working order.

Because the new hip is near the soft tissues of the pelvis, your urinary tract might cease its everyday work, too. This occurs more often among men than women, especially among men with an enlarged prostate gland. It is known as **urinary retention**, and can be found in up to a third of patients. To help men a urinary catheter is put up the penis into the bladder. Women might find that when they are lying down in bed it is difficult to pass urine, and later, when they get up and walk about, the problem diminishes. But urinary retention might be made worse by discovering an infection in the urinary tract that was not observed before the operation: antibiotics will probably solve that problem.

In bed men are given a flask into which they urinate and a pan to use for defecation; women sit on a bedpan. Using a bedpan can be very awkward and off-putting no matter how much you feel you need to use it.

I felt that I was very fortunate because no problems arose. I had had an operation many years earlier, knew the routine intimately, and had long since discarded the embarrassment that goes with the need to urinate and defecate with others nearby and perhaps having nurses clear up afterwards.

I had a bottle to use for urine. On Wednesday morning, thirty-six hours after the operation, I needed to use the toilet and was given a stainless steel bedpan. I grabbed the triangle above me, sat on the bedpan, used it, removed the pan, placed it and its contents on the bedside table, and put the bedpan into an enormous paper bag. All this was done in five minutes. Strange as it might seem, this was quite a rewarding effort. When the nurse came to take away the bedpan she too was surprised. Thereafter I did not use a bedpan. Later that day I was told that I would be getting up soon and would be using the lavatory.

Ernst's medical experience and technical knowledge made urinating and defecation and their attendant problems easy to manage.

"I did have some urinary retention after the first operation. They had an eight-hourly drip of solution going in, and I was drinking and eating. So I wanted to pass urine all the time, but I had to have an injection of **Urecoline** to enable me to pass urine. I learned from that, and for the second operation I insisted that the drip be slowed down and removed, and I restricted my drinking. I had to have a **suppository** for the bowels the first time, but by the second time I'd learned."

Charles had a similar problem.

"I didn't pee very well for the first night. They were going to rescue me with a catheter, but I came good in the end. Bowels functioned after five days. I think I had two goes and a pee sitting on the bed, and then after that I was OK. They told me that's the turning point of the whole exercise."

Years later Mario could still remember the inhibition associated with urinating. For him, the physical inhibition was the central feeling.

"I can remember the feeling that I really did want to urinate but it couldn't happen, and didn't happen for twenty-four hours, or just twelve waking hours. But having the sensation of wanting to pass water and not being able to do it makes you realise there's been chemical changes and other things. Perhaps those normal processes have deliberately been inhibited, and are a carry-over from the operation. That's the way I felt about it."

Terri had to urinate, but nothing happened to her.

"I knew I had to go to the loo, but they stuck me on a pan, and they had to run the tap to try and get me to go. All the staff kept going out to the loo! It worked on everyone else, not me."

Betty, a much older woman than Terri, found the difficulties and indignity of using the bedpan most distressing.

"I really was very well. I had no problem with eating. The only problem I had was getting on to a bedpan. That was awful. The male nurse had to do all that. Lift me. I had no strength at all. And my back was bad, too."

Bernard was just as distressed as Betty about defecating in a bed because he felt deeply how offensive it would be for the nurse.

"Bedpans! I held on for five days. Lucky I did because I got diarrhoea on the day. I said to the young nurse that morning, 'Well, you'd have to be the luckiest nurse around, you know.' She asked me why, and I explained to her that she would have been in and out with the pan every five minutes."

Mario worried that as days went past he couldn't move his bowels, and that when he did the stench would be overwhelming. Next time he was well prepared.

"I knew that I was taking food in. When was it going to go? Who was going to be the unfortunate person who had to help out? That is a very personal situation. You know that you can't relieve yourself, and you know that somebody's going to have to do it. I think the staff were good about that. I think next time I'll take a little bottle of perfume and put it beside the bed and just leave it for the nurse who has that job."

Caring for a patient's toilet needs is part of the nurse's normal role, and is done with understanding and thoughtfulness, not embarrassment or revulsion. However humiliated you might feel at first, be assured that this feeling will quickly pass as the work of getting better becomes the focus of your attention.

Dislocation

There you are, on your back, breathing through a plastic oxygen mask, the triangular Charnley abduction pillow between your ankles, and nurses telling you plainly that you must lie on your back, not on your side, and not to think of turning over or trying to cross your legs or turn your feet inwards.

The risk of dislocation is quite slim — between five and thirty in a thousand. Dislocation occurs because the tone of the muscle around the hip is poor, or because your surgeon has made a mistake due to lack of experience. Your surgeon's reputation depends on the success of your operation, and, among the complications that can arise with hip surgery, dislocation is most embarrassing. It also hurts. So the surgeon, the nurses, the hospital, and you have a great investment in the new hip not dislocating. If it does, chances are that it will not dislocate again.

It is your responsibility to be sure that you follow the nurses' and the physiotherapist's advice never to cross your legs or bend your hip more than 90 degrees. Despite this, there are a very few people who dislocate more than once, and they might have to wear a special device or have another operation on their new hip (a revision). The operation is difficult and might not be successful.

Dislocation is always a possibility, and it is there for the rest of your life. Be advised: take special note of what your surgeon and nurses say, and do as you are told. You will know if you dislocate your new hip by the return of pain.

Infection

Occasionally you will be given an injection of antibiotics to reduce the likelihood of infection. The chances of infection are very low: about one in a hundred for deep infection, and slightly more for an infection on the surface of your wound. Some surgeons reject the distinction between shallow and deep infections.

An infected wound will feel hot, and the medical staff will see that it is red. It will be dealt with quickly. Deep infection does not respond to treatment so rapidly and is generally hard to eradicate. In the hospital, and especially the operating theatre, sterile methods are used with antibiotics and a special air flow system to prevent infection. If infection does occur, another operation might be necessary. And there is no guarantee; in fact the revision operation attracts a higher chance of infection than the original hip replacement.

Blood flow

Close attention is given to the blood flow in the days immediately after the operation. Blood clotting is a risk at this time. Swellings, blood pressure falling, blood count changing, bleeding from the wound, and a curious use of the autologous blood donation all occurred in my informants' experiences.

Blood clots

When you wake up, chances are that you will find your legs in either full-length or half-length white TED (thromboembolic deterrent) or DVT (deep vein thrombosis) stockings. They are used to reduce the probability of a blood clot forming in the leg and finding its way to the lung, where it could be fatal. Not all surgeons use the stockings, because their value is not securely known or understood. So if you find yourself without white stockings, your surgeon is using some other technique, such as a regular injection near the stomach, to offset the chances of blood clots affecting the success of the surgery.

Deep vein thrombosis is more common among female than male patients. It seems that if you are older than 70 you have slightly more than a 50 per cent chance of deep vein thrombosis if you do not have the white stockings. So wear them, and if you want to complain about how uncomfortable they surely are, do so, but be assured that complaining will not help. You will probably be expected to wear them for the next six weeks.

Ernst was adamant about the use of white stockings, but found that perhaps they did not need to be full-length.

> "For the second operation I only had the shorter stockings, and even that was only for four weeks. I'd much rather have to wear them than have a deep vein thrombosis. You could die quickly."

The use of white stockings was not common when Tess had her first operation fifteen years ago. Also in those days there were none of the now-commonplace tests for blood clotting. Eight years later she did wear the stockings and took warfarin tablets to prevent blood clots. The second time her condition was complicated by bruises, which seemed to her to have arisen because of the way she was operated on.

"I did not have the long stockings for the first operation. No blood tests or tablets for blood clotting. I was on warfarin for a short time in hospital. The second time I had trouble with the warfarin because I got a big, massive bruise on this leg. He had operated with me mostly on my side. I had the spinal anaesthetic for the second operation. I remember distinctly him saying: 'Tilt it over a wee bit.' I heard all this as I went in. It was a very good spinal. I certainly didn't feel a thing from the waist down. I was awake. And he said, 'I want her tilted that way.' So I was half on my side, and there must have been pressure on the leg. There was a massive bruise. When he came to see me I said, 'I've got this massive bruise on my leg. What happened?' And he looked at it, and said, 'No more warfarin.' I'd been on warfarin, but I didn't know I'd been on it. That was the second op. I don't remember any warfarin in the first operation at all."

Blood pressure falls suddenly

Doug went through the shock of finding his blood pressure fall and saw the importance of a supply of his own blood for an emergency after the operation.

"About half past eight, night time, everything seemed to be fine. Then my blood pressure started to drop away and got to be a real worry. They started to phone around, and by one o'clock I had in attendance resident specialists, another doctor, and various nursing staff. They turned me over. The wound was bleeding. They decided they would give me another litre of my remaining autologous blood. They also gave me something else, another fluid. They were at me all night, checking me, the blood pressure, and the wound. The wound was bleeding, but it wasn't the cause of the low blood pressure. The cause of the low blood pressure was my reaction to the epidural."

Blood count is too low

Charles was surprised to find his haemoglobin level was too low. Normally it would be between 12 and 18 g per 100 ml of blood.

"My blood count went right down to about eight in the hospital. I got very ill, and so I was on all sorts of iron stuff, and spinach and iron tablets. And by the time I left the hospital it was back to about ten, I think. But it didn't get up to anything like normal until the last blood test, which was in six weeks."

The wound bleeds

Bernard did not understand why the wound appeared to be bleeding all the time he was in hospital.

"The wound wept. It had clips on it. They took the draining tubes out after about two days. It just oozed away until the day before I came home. I'd get the dressing changed three or four times a day. It is amazing how different surgeons have different ideas. This surgeon of mine wouldn't even let the nurses put a tape on it to hold it there. It had to be just the dressing and the white stockings over the top."

Unusual use of the autologous blood donation

Ernst wanted to accelerate his rate of recovery. He understood the effect of adding his own blood to his body soon after the operation. He persuaded his surgeon that it would be best if he were given a blood transfusion, which, under normal circumstances, both knew would not be regarded as necessary. The unused blood can be kept at the blood bank for only thirty days.

"I gave two units of blood. If you don't use your two units of blood, and they're not given to you, they're just thrown out. They don't go back to the blood bank. My surgeon said my first operation had been almost bloodless. I had no units of blood during the operation, and he gave me one immediately post-op. And I said to him the next day, 'I've got a unit of blood sitting there. It seems to me if I had that, it'd give me a bit more energy to get moving.' He said, 'Oh, you don't need it.' I said, 'Well, it's only going to be wasted. Can I have it?' So he gave it to me, and I think that enabled me to have more energy. They say they won't transfuse unless you're haemoglobin's above, in the old terms, 9 grams, albeit that your normal level might be 11–13 grams. I say, if my blood level's 9, and I've got a unit sitting there that I've donated, and 9 is still 2 points below the normal levels, then it seems to me, my recovery is likely to be speeded up. I'll have more energy if I have extra blood. I would have the oxygen-carrying capacity back again. I also wonder if that was a factor in my recovering faster than some other people, too. If your haemoglobin's only 9, and if you're used to having a haemoglobin of 12 or 13, you're going to be tired, and lacking in energy and listless. I was revving and ready to go straight away. I didn't want to stay in bed."

Nevertheless, there are advantages to a patient having a reduced haemoglobin level, especially if the surgeon thinks it might decrease the likelihood of a blood clot.

Swellings appear

Terri thought she might have dislocated her new hip because beside it was a enormous swelling that did not seem to go away.

> "I had a big pouch of swelling hanging there, and it subsided within five days of being home. That was uncomfortable, but I didn't know from that uncomfortable feeling whether I'd dislocated the hip, because it felt so odd. I'd known that was a possibility."

Terri's swelling was caused by the shock of surgery. It would normally diminish over time.

Conclusion

The shock to your body of a hip replacement operation is severe and requires expert attention for few days. What medical staff anticipate usually takes place. However clear are their expectations, the staff know that each patient is both a special medical case and a unique person who recovers at their own rate in their own way. For this reason you will be given close care when you emerge from the operating room.

I was fortunate because only one thing seemed to go wrong. My stomach became bloated for a day. Attention was given to it immediately. My informants endured a catalogue of problems that I did not know could arise. They were associated with sleeping, pain, minor discomforts, unusual responses to the anaesthetic, eating difficulties, concerns about the toilet, blood pressure scares, irritating white stockings, and swellings. Under careful supervision these problems were not allowed to worsen and impede recovery in the next few days.

6

Recovery — after the first few days

Two days after the operation you will be expected to get up and use a walking frame to cross the room. Unless there is still much fluid coming from the wound, your drain tubes will be taken out, and your painkiller and sickness tablets will be reduced. Your blood will have been monitored for haemoglobin. If the count is low you might have to take some iron tablets or even have a blood transfusion. As a precaution, your surgeon might have the hip X-rayed just to establish a benchmark against which later developments can be assessed.

On the third day you could be back to your normal diet, and able to walk about twenty paces with the frame and even to sit in a chair for a while. If you need no blood transfusion your drip will have been removed. Painkiller and anti-sickness tablets will still be used, and you could have an injection to reduce the possibility of deep vein thrombosis. On day 4 you will be given underarm or elbow crutches to replace your frame. You will still be using painkiller and anti-sickness tablets or injections. If necessary you might discuss convalescence at home with an occupational therapist or social worker.

Over the next three days your recovery will quicken. The painkillers will not seem so necessary, but treatment to limit the chances of deep vein thrombosis will continue unchanged. You will begin to feel more and more responsible for your recovery.

By the eighth day you will be shown how to go up and down steps, put on your shoes, and pick up fallen items. You are almost ready to go home. In the next two or three days your wound will be attended to. If your wound was stitched, stitches will be taken out; any staples will be removed. And if things have gone as expected, on day 10 you will leave hospital.

This is a common pattern of recovery based on everyday experience in hospital. So in the pattern of recovery, the expected steps and the timing are a guide, not a prescription for recovery. Patients recover at their own pace.

From walking frame to crutches

I was given precise instructions about getting myself from a lying position to the edge of the bed where the walking frame was waiting. I was watched very closely indeed. I raised myself with the left hand, gripped the triangle above my head, and moved myself forward down to the middle of the bed. My right hand was placed in the centre of the bed. I leaned on the right arm and slowly sat up straight; then, as I turned to the left, my left leg, the operated one, gradually slipped off the bed. I turned slowly to the left, supported myself on my hands, and leaned forward over the edge of the bed. Meanwhile the nurse, under the eye of the physiotherapist, had placed a walking frame in front of me. I leaned forward over my feet, gripped the walking frame, stood, and walked across the room. Sounds easy, but it was quite an effort.

Late that evening, again under close supervision, I managed to raise myself and make it to the other side of the room. An hour or so later I crossed the outside corridor. That was about forty-eight hours after the operation. Recovery had begun. Each day I walked a little further. After three days or so the walking frame gave way to two elbow crutches. Two days later I was given one crutch. Eight days after the operation I was expected to go home. I was happy to leave, but there was no one to drive me home, so I discharged myself three days later.

I left hospital dressed in a pair of light-weight cotton slacks pulled over the white TED/DVT stockings, a sports shirt, and the Velcro-tabbed shoes. One elbow crutch steadied me. I received a detailed account of all the costs of the operation and stay in hospital, and was glad that I had full health insurance cover. The chair that I would use in the toilet at home was put into the back of the station wagon. The two elbow crutches fitted easily across the back seat.

Among the patients around you it becomes clear that the recovery rate varies. The character, style, preferences, and expectations of surgeons are not the same. Doug noticed great differences in recovery rate between the people in his ward, as well as the different approaches of the surgeons.

> "In forty-eight hours I was sitting on the side of the bed. I could put weight on the feet and use a frame, then elbow crutches. I found that each specialist has a different way of treating people. Maybe it's your age. A man with a hip replacement had been there nine days and hadn't put his foot down on the ground. He was a bit older, but he was very fit. They were talking about even longer periods when I went home. I was out in nine days. But there were people who were in for the fourteen days. And some of them were going into sort of remedial care. Everyone was older than me, except two footballers who were coming in to get their knees done."

Doug and I followed the expected pattern of recovery, but others took longer than us to get out of bed and walk. For example, Charles said:

> "I got up on the sixth day, with a walking frame, walked to the window, with people on either side of me, and then got back into bed. That was enough. And then I used two elbow crutches two or three days later. I was thirteen days in hospital. By the time I came out I could sort of walk, with crutches and with considerable difficulty."

Mario remembered few details, but always had the impression that the recovery was well structured.

> "I was up in perhaps forty-eight hours, with a walking frame. I think there was a very deliberate staged process. I can remember a week afterwards walking tentatively around one circuit of the ward."

Bernard spent four days in bed. Terri was out of bed on her third day but found the walking frame did not suit her. She preferred to get out of bed in her own way, rather than do as her physiotherapist instructed.

"I found getting up using my own arm was the easiest thing to do in bed. They offered that little triangle above, but I didn't use it. The very first day I got out of bed I was with the physio, and it was wonderful to have that shower. I didn't really like the frame, although the sticks wouldn't have been enough support in those early few days. With the frame, you have to use your chest muscles to hold on. Using the frame I got a rhythm that I was happy with, but the physio didn't like it, and she wanted me to keep the frame further out, and I didn't like that. I wanted to do it my way, which I knew I was comfortable with, and I felt safe with. But she didn't feel good about that. So I didn't work with the frame very well. I was only on that frame for a few days anyhow. I took my own underarm crutches into hospital with me because I'd had them from the previous surgery. I stayed two weeks."

On one hand Betty also felt that she had been pushed into the process of recovery, but on the other hand she appreciated the need to get on with it. She used a frame with wheels, later used sticks, and never used crutches at all.

"After a couple of days they get you up and make you go and have a shower. I don't remember ever being washed in bed. I felt it was very right that they should do this because people would feel that they were invalids, and these days you're not."

Nell compared herself with other patients and felt she was slower in her recovery. She got up in the second week rather than on the second day of her stay in hospital.

"I wasn't as quick as a lot of people. I don't think it did any harm because I had almost two weeks in hospital, and then I had another two weeks at a rehabilitation hospital."

Tess's recovery was different again.

"On the fourth day I was up. A little on the fourth day. I stayed in for the full fortnight. I used elbow crutches for a bit, but I came out on two sticks. I came straight home."

Physiotherapy

Twice every day a nurse would remind me to do the physiotherapist's board exercises and ensure that I followed the strict rules of recovery.

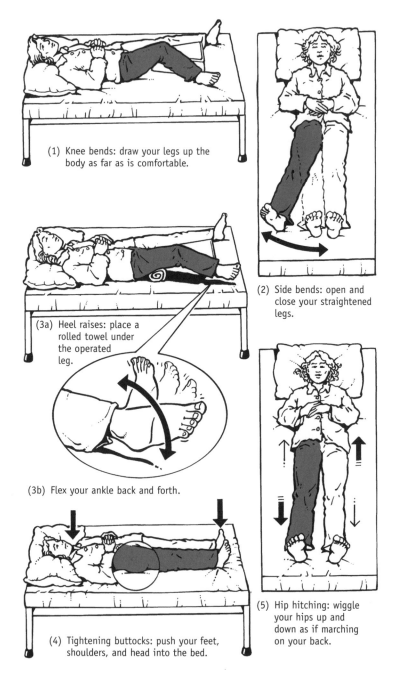

(1) Knee bends: draw your legs up the body as far as is comfortable.

(2) Side bends: open and close your straightened legs.

(3a) Heel raises: place a rolled towel under the operated leg.

(3b) Flex your ankle back and forth.

(4) Tightening buttocks: push your feet, shoulders, and head into the bed.

(5) Hip hitching: wiggle your hips up and down as if marching on your back.

Figure 6: Five exercises to help you recover after the operation.

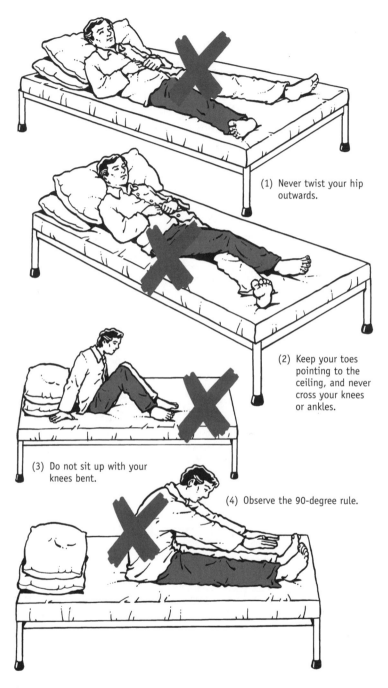

(1) Never twist your hip outwards.

(2) Keep your toes pointing to the ceiling, and never cross your knees or ankles.

(3) Do not sit up with your knees bent.

(4) Observe the 90-degree rule.

Figure 7: Lying in bed.

The first involved drawing one's legs up the body as far as was comfortable (knee bends); then opening and closing straightened legs (side bends); flexing the ankles back and forth with a rolled towel under the thigh of the operated leg (heel raises); tightening the muscles of the buttocks; and hitching the hips up and down as if marching while on one's back (hip-hitching).

The first three exercises are usually done with a slippery board under the heels to help them slide easily. In the beginning I was expected to do these exercises twice a day five times, later ten times, and eventually twenty to thirty times. I found that the slippery board was not necessary because my heels slid easily across the sheets.

Strict rules govern where you may place your legs. They were apart because the abduction pillow was always between my legs, except when exercising. I was told never to twist my new hip; when lying on my back, I must point my toes ceiling-wards to prevent myself from rolling my legs. This I found hard to remember, and often the nurse would tweak my left foot as she passed the end

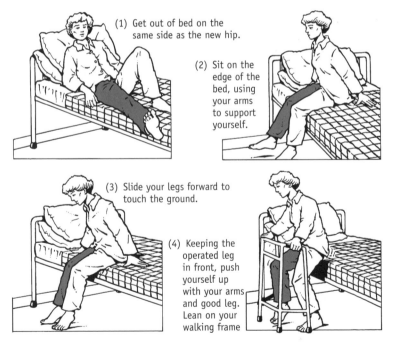

(1) Get out of bed on the same side as the new hip.

(2) Sit on the edge of the bed, using your arms to support yourself.

(3) Slide your legs forward to touch the ground.

(4) Keeping the operated leg in front, push yourself up with your arms and good leg. Lean on your walking frame

Figure 8: Getting out of bed.

(1), (2), (3) Sit in a chair with arms, with your crutch nearby, and stand slowly with the operated leg in front of you.

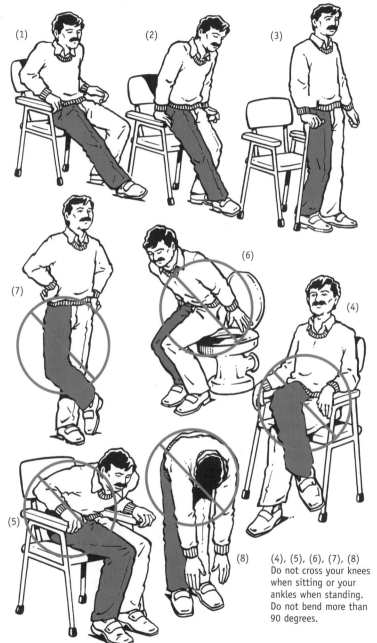

(4), (5), (6), (7), (8)
Do not cross your knees when sitting or your ankles when standing. Do not bend more than 90 degrees.

Figure 9: Sitting and walking.

of the bed. Everyone insisted that I never bend my hip more than 90 degrees. When getting out of bed alone I was told to do so only on the side of the new hip. Finally the golden rule: never cross the legs in bed, sitting or standing.

These rules seem to come naturally at first. To get out of bed I would sit on the edge of the bed, support myself with my arms, slide my legs forward on to the ground, with the operated leg way out in front of me, and push myself up with the good leg. This skill did not take long to develop. To sit in a chair, one slightly higher than most, with high arms, I would back into the chair, keep my operated leg as straight as I could, place the crutches within easy reach, and lower myself slowly into the chair by the arms. The natural movement seemed to be to keep the operated leg straight. In time I found that with it straight there was no trouble bending forward a little more each day, and eventually it was easy to pick up fallen items without using the extension arm.

Doug had the same rules to follow and the same exercises.

> "You swing to the side as much as was comfortable and various other things, morning and afternoon. And the nurses used to set you up for that."

Bernard kept his exercise list, brought it home, and showed me a copy. He chanted:

> "Don't let your leg roll inwards, don't cross your legs, don't bend your hip above 90 degrees."

Charles took the physiotherapist seriously, approached her exercise program with great vigour, and, although the program felt dull and uncomfortable, was pleased to discover it was most helpful.

> "The physio was very robust in her approach. I took the view that you've only got one chance to get it right, and I wouldn't do anything to contribute to the chances being diminished. I found some of the exercises very boring and very painful. But I used to spend thirty-five minutes on them by the time I left hospital."

By contrast, Terri was not happy with her physiotherapy because it tired her, and she felt the physiotherapist did not approach the work with her needs in mind.

"When I did walk, it was painful. I'd walk to the toilet and come back exhausted. Each day I had the physio come every morning after I'd had my shower. Even though I was still in bed, she'd give a little instruction to tighten my leg, move my toes, or do whatever I can. Later I said to the physio, 'You're coming at the wrong time. I'm exhausted. I don't want to get up and go for a walk now. I've just been in my shower for a half an hour, and I've just done my walk.' When I got the bill, I thought, 'Damn her. I'm paying for her, and she comes when it suits her. She's charging me pretty impressive fees to come when it suited her and not me.' "

Because she did not want to tire herself, Tess paced her recovery through its stages. At first she found the physiotherapist's exercises were difficult and could bring no vigour to them. Her recovery began with exercises in bed for three days before she got up.

"The exercises were to pull the legs up, over, out, and back. Then I would just gently draw the legs up the bed. I found that was difficult. I would like to have done it differently, but she wouldn't let me. More than anything, they wanted the abductor muscles on the inside of the leg moving some time before you stood up. I think I stood on the fourth day. I got out of bed with only the physio there and with a walking frame. I could go to the bathroom with the walking frame on my own about the fifth or sixth day."

Unlike Tess, Ernst, who left hospital on day 5, worked vigorously at the task of getting better, far too quickly for his physiotherapist's satisfaction. She was concerned about dislocation.

"If you were a surgeon and you had some patient who'd gone ahead too fast and dislocated, you'd learn to be conservative. I remember the physio catching me, after my first operation, in the physio area where I was doing a training session on the steps. I was just going up and down the steps, up and down the steps, and then doing a circuit of work because I'm used to training like that. She said, 'Look, I can see you're doing it fine, but you're not supposed to train at it. Once you can do it you don't have to worry any more.' She restrained me. She was right. I was lucky to have a surgeon who trusted me not to be silly and knew what was happening."

His surgeon allowed him a great deal of autonomy in achieving freedom of movement. Ernst did not fear dislocation so much as heterotopic ossification (unusual bone growth around the hip joint), which can limit movement and tends to occur more often among heavy than light people. Ernst had a very large frame.

"After so long I was determined to have the freedom of movement in the hips. The surgeon put me on one of the early anti-inflammatories. It is supposed to be good at limiting that ossification. So I stayed on that for four weeks, post-operatively, and indeed my movement is just fantastic."

You must expect to be watched closely as you recover, add to your strength and mobility, and be encouraged towards the goal of independence; but you will be restrained to avoid accidents and the threat of dislocation. Probably you will be supervised best, and know you are progressing well, when the nurses begin to ignore you. This is a good sign of growing independence.

Useful items for becoming independent

You will be allowed to go home when you are well along the path to independence. The decision is taken by the surgeon. You will be discharged when you can get out of bed without a nurse being there to hold you, go to the toilet and shower alone, and walk a reasonable distance with one or two sticks or crutches.

In hospital you will learn useful skills and the value of various items to make life easier. Because you may not stoop or bend beyond 90 degrees, you will have problems with putting on your shoes, socks or stockings, picking up dropped items, washing your feet, showering, and sitting on the conventional toilet. Many of these problems will be quite unfamiliar to you, although you will have been told about them before entering hospital.

After I had been shown how to use the walking frame I took a shower alone on the third day. At first it was difficult and slow. I held on to whatever seemed secure, and I moved cautiously. In two days I became quite adept. Nevertheless, drying my back in the confined space of the shower room was always difficult.

Mario had his first shower after about a week. Nell had hers about half way through her two-week stay. Bernard had his first shower much sooner in a spacious recess with enough room for a wheelchair and, like Doug, learned the value of the extension arm in the shower.

"There was a seat there for me to sit on if I needed to. There was no soap on a rope, but they had plenty of handrails and racks and other things. I had a picker-up thing [extension arm]. I dropped the face washer one morning. You can't bend down to pick it up. I'd got my picker-up thing there on the bench beside me, so I picked it up."

Doug had been told little about the conditions under which he would recover. The hospital had no pre-admission clinic. The information he did get meant nothing to him until the operation was over and recovery had begun. Like many of my informants, he was not aware of the useful items available to help him gain independence.

"Although they provided me with an information sheet, you don't know what a lot of it is about. You don't know what is that sock puller-onner [sock helper or sock aid], and long pliers-like grippers, like callipers [extension arm or extension hand], and other things you can get to give you independence. Basically independence is what it's all about. I found out a lot of other things I would have done differently. I didn't realise how simple these sock puller-onners are, so simple that you can make them out of cardboard. Or you could use a pair of long-handled barbecue tongs in place of the grippers [extension arm]. Better than those expensive things that you'd probably never use again. I had a shoehorn of some length. That's OK mainly for putting on slippers. A portable mirror was handy, too."

Terri was so fascinated by her extension arm that she destroyed the first one!

"I bought one of those calliper things [extension arm]. It was funny when I bought that. I was by myself when it arrived, and I pulled it apart, pulled the whole string out of the middle of it, and I totally wrecked it. The people I bought it from were really good. They just came the next day, delivered another one, and took it back to rethread it and fix it. I had no use for a long shoehorn, or soap on a rope either."

From his brother Bernard found the Velcro-tabbed shoes that I had discovered and now swears that they are the most useful shoes for someone who is not allowed to bend beyond the 90-degree angle.

"My brother had these shoes. He said they're the only things to have. Now I can pick them up of a morning and sit on the bed, pick them up by the tongue with my tongs, slip my foot in, and pull the Velcro straps across the tongues."

Betty was uncomfortable in bed.

"But I did feel that I needed the piece of sheepskin. I found that the backs of my heels got very rough and almost blistery. They did provide sheepskin. That was very necessary, as well as the pillow between my knees."

Being nursed

Being cared for in hospital leaves different impressions. Early impressions arise from specific personal help with the toilet, one's immediate comfort in bed, the control of pain, and sleeping problems, while others are related to a general and diffuse feeling of well-being. The most notable change is that you feel better. At the same time you reach a turning point where your independence is evident, and the nurses become aware that they are not needed so often. You do not have to say anything to them. They can see you getting better, they tell each other about you, and you find you do not need, or get, the close attention that was required, demanded, and offered when you first came from the operating theatre. Before you reach that turning point you might enjoy little luxuries reminiscent of childhood. On the other hand you might be in pain, not from the operation directly, but from the moves necessary to nurse you properly. Being nursed is a rewarding, pleasurable, and sometimes positively infantilising experience; other times it can be quite frustrating because of incompetence and apparent carelessness.

Nell remembered a moment of paradise when one nurse 'washed my hair the day before I left, which was heaven'. Bernard found the nursing was exceptionally good, and obviously enjoyed it.

"They would turn me over to wash me, and it felt good, actually, because I could get on to my side. They call it a 'log roll' with the pillow between your legs, and they roll you over. I used to pull the pillow between my legs. I thought it was great to lie on my side for a while. I didn't sweat on my back because I was on sheepskin all the time. That was supplied. Not being able to sleep and having to lie on your back all the time meant your back gets sore. Every so often the nurses used to give it a rub. That was the best part of recovering. After about seven or eight days the physio got me a chair to put beside the bed, and I started moving around. I was getting out three or four times through the night and just sitting in the chair right outside the night nurse's office, opposite the door to the ward. They'd see me sitting there and they'd bring me a cup of tea. It was quite good. Nurses took the white stockings off each day. After the shower they put them back on."

A quite different story came from Tess, herself a nurse of many years experience, who was also hurt by the nurses. She was obviously so unhappy that one day her charge nurse intervened. It is necessary for you to lie flat for a period twice each day so that the muscle on the top of your thigh is stretched sufficiently.

"After lunch each day they made the bed flatter and lengthened me out so that I had to pull on this muscle. I had to have half an hour of that. One night I wasn't sleeping because the leg was quite painful. When the nurse came in I said: 'I don't know why. I haven't done anything different today, but my leg is quite painful.' Quite a young girl, she said: 'Well, you can't have anything.' I said: 'I know I can't have anything for the pain, but I am just wondering why, because I haven't done anything different today.' A bit later on a more senior nurse came in, and she said: 'You're not asleep yet.' 'No,' I said. 'My leg's painful. I don't know why.' 'You're too flat,' she said. And she wound the bed up. Then she brought me in some sleeping pills. And when I woke up the next morning the sleeping pills were there. As soon as they had put the bed up it had taken off the pressure, and I went to sleep. The younger nurse didn't pick that up. The senior nurse did."

To her annoyance Terri found that her hospital was being renovated, and the staff were not familiar with the new communication system.

"And they had these tinny buzzers that went ting, ting, ting. These buzzers would drive me mad. In the end I learned to switch off. On one occasion in the early days [of my recovery] I was on a bedpan. And I had the buzzer ringing for twenty minutes, waiting for a nurse to come and take it. She eventually forgot. They weren't accustomed to hearing the bell."

Terri had waited a long time for her used bedpan to be taken away because the young trainee had been so busy she had forgotten her.

"She was a trainee nurse. She came in, and she tipped half the contents over me. I was furious. I said I wanted a bed wash and a change. Everything and now! I was wild with her. I had the hospital matron come and apologise to me that day. The length of time it takes for them to come and see you once you ring the bell! If you wait until you're in pain, then they come, and they've got to go away and get their keys and another person to administer a medication. This whole thing can take half an hour, and you're getting in worse pain. Then you've got to wait another half an hour or twenty minutes for the stuff to start working. I know they're probably busy, but that's just a real inconvenience."

Although she was moved from room to room during the renovations at the hospital, Terri also recalled being well looked after.

"On the second day I was finally in a room of my own! And then they had the X-ray machine come in and do the X-ray. They brought the machine to me! I did get up on the third day, with a walking frame. The nurses were wonderfully helpful with the skin rashes."

However, Terri did not like her stay in hospital because of the uncaring nursing and the pain of being turned over.

"You're just going to hurt when they turn you. You're at their mercy, totally at their mercy, and they're tipping you over. 'I hope you catch me here!' I said. Yes, it's all unsettling."

When the operation that Helen needed was no longer available at a public hospital, she had had to attend a private hospital three years ago. Recently, when she returned to the same private hospital for another operation, she soon became aware of the reduced services.

"The good experience about the hospital was that the nursing staff were all the same from three years ago, and that makes a huge difference. There's been cost-cutting, I've noticed. And the ratio of staff to patients is a bit less than it was three years ago. They were all very good."

Helen had nothing but praise for the nurses who helped her.

"I had a great relationship with the nurses. I really got on with them very well, because I was there for so long and knew them."

Doug thought in retrospect that the nursing staff was good to him.

"Nursing was fine. The whole staff, doctors, and food. No complaints about that. And you get to know a lot of people by the time you leave. A young female physio came. She was very, very helpful."

Like Terri, Fred also was not pleased with the service of incompetent young nurses.

"The nurses were very young and they didn't know what they were doing. I had one older nurse who knew what a patient needed. But the young nurses had no feeling at all for a patient. They hurt me each day they rolled me over on my side to prevent bed sores. I knew they had to do it, but they didn't know how to do it without hurting me. And they didn't care much, either. I wouldn't go back to that hospital."

Mario also had an unhappy experience of clumsy nursing, confined to only one nurse, but he was pleased to be nursed so well by others.

"There was one particular nurse who was insensitive. I think that's the worst thing a nurse can be — insensitive. I used to like getting my backside rubbed in the wee hours of the morning. They sprinkled something, a soothing chemical, calamine lotion, on my back."

Nell was much slower than most to recover. She felt pushed at first, and found efforts to prevent her getting a rash distressingly uncomfortable, but in time her nursing became all that she could ask for.

"I didn't want to get up when they wanted because I wasn't comfortable. I just didn't feel I was ready. When they turned me over they were very good, always three or four nurses. They put the sides up, and they tell you how to get your arms across first and hold on, and then they'd say 'One-two-three and go' and push. I dreaded that. It didn't prevent me getting a rash on my back. After a few days I did get a rash on my back, but that went. They got calamine. But it wasn't through lack of care."

Curiosity about the operation

Most of us are ignorant about the operation largely because of the ambivalence it inspires. It is a brutal and violent activity, yet at the same time it is enormously valued for the relief from pain its brings and the increasing mobility it confers. On television the operating theatre is a stage for entertainment and horror, the setting for life and death, romance, tests, bitter jealousies, and unending human conflicts for young and old. It is not surprising that the ambivalent imagery emerging from the operating theatre creates curiosity about details of surgery. This curiosity about surgery is due to the fact that it is both invasive and intimate. In an operating theatre people are going to do things to you, and you don't know what.

Before my operation, I did not want to know. After my operation, I was mildly curious. I did not want to ask the surgeon, largely because I did not want too much information, and felt I was intruding on sacred ground. In a few days I learned a little about the operation. No one volunteered information about what had happened. It was only from a conversation I overheard between nurses that I knew my anaesthetic had been a general anaesthetic and that my new hip had been cementless.

Terri and Helen, whose lives were dominated by serious problems with rheumatoid arthritis, were far more curious about the operation. Terri's sister, herself a nurse, told her enough to put to rest much curiosity about the operation.

"When she came in to see me, four or five days after the surgery, I wanted to know explicitly what they do when you're under the anaesthetic, and so she told me in every detail. I didn't want to know before, but I needed to know after. The doctor has said that the pain is caused by the weight displacement coming through the prosthesis into your own bone. That was extraordinarily intense pain, and it lasted right through the time I was in hospital, even up to the day before I was coming home. I was having heat packs for that."

Helen also learned about her operation from the nurses at the hospital.

"I was in this private hospital three years ago for the right side, and I went back three months ago to have the left done. This time I had a bone graft, and that takes an enormous length of time to grow back to be solid bone. The nurses were fairly good at telling me about the structure of the bone graft. They take bone from the **bone bank**, grind it up, basically in a mortar and pestle, then remove the impurities, build a wire frame, and then bang it in really hard. It's a bit like reinforced concrete. The nurses used the cheesecake base as an analogy. It holds well and good, but as soon as you put any weight on it, it could easily crumble to bits. So there's a fair bit of fear with a bone graft. It can easily shatter. The bone is growing around the prosthesis to strengthen my pelvis because it's small and worn out, and they can't just whip the whole thing out and replace it with a plastic one. That'll probably come."

Pain, discomfort, and weariness

I found moving in bed no trouble. However, for some informants moving was far from painless. In time, pain would diminish into discomfort and eventually go, but when doing daily chores of washing oneself and turning over in bed it was never gone, especially for Nell.

"Pain came with the moving, and the bathing and sitting up. You slide down quite a bit in bed, and when you have to sit up to have a meal, it takes a bit of agonising and getting up. And I didn't have much strength; that was the thing. I hadn't played tennis for twenty-five years, so I have no muscles in my arms to help me along. I really noticed that. It would've been a good idea if I'd done some sort of exercises beforehand. Being turned over was the worst part every day. So was washing your back and getting you on to your side. I found that extremely painful. They'd always give painkillers about twenty minutes before that happened."

Tess was surprised to find that she was in as much pain as ever after her first operation, especially when doing the physio-therapist's exercises.

"The first time I didn't know if it was going to be very painful afterwards, and it was. I wasn't conscious of the wound being painful. It's a very long incision. I was distressed to find the right leg muscle still in pain. I had everything that I went in with. Every movement from the second day I found very painful. And one day when the physio left I was almost in tears. My surgeon came in, and asked, 'What's up?' 'I've got all the same symptoms that I came in with,' I said. 'I've been through all this. And I've still got all the same symptoms. I've still got all this pain in the side and everything. It's when I move, and it's in every movement.' He said: 'Well, you will for a bit. It'll go.' Then he sent me down for an X-ray just in case things weren't right. I really had sailed through it very well until then. After that it went well."

Terri also found that the pain from physiotherapy was not what she had anticipated.

"What was so unexpected was this pain in my leg, which was as bad as the hip. It was that top muscle of the leg, and in fact I still get it. And whenever the physio would try to move my leg outwards, it was excruciating. It was worse than my hip."

Apart from the pain, which diminished in a few days, I had discomforts, some of which lasted almost as long as the stay in hospital. Although I was able to wash myself in the shower, sitting on a special seat, and use the toilet, on a slightly raised seat, I found it hard to dry my body. I also perspired in bed, which led to a rash developing on my back. It itched and irritated me for the length of my stay in hospital, but very little could be done about it. My back soon became a mass of tiny pimple-like irritations. Finally I got some relief with a medicated talcum powder.

Mario had back pain, and he too developed a bed rash, which wasn't pleasant but was expected. Nurses would come to bathe him in the small hours because they were too busy during the day.

As her rate of recovery began to increase Nell felt better, but she could see that her recovery was much slower than that of others.

"I found it rather difficult. I got a bit sick of this business of lying with your legs spread with a pillow in between. Of course you really need sleeping tablets every night. I was a bit slow. They wanted me out of bed before I wanted to be out. They'd sit me in the chair, and I'd be very uncomfortable and I'd always get back quickly. Other people gave me the impression that they were a little quicker at walking on crutches to the door and back. But I was very afraid of my balance. They got me up with a frame and a nurse on either side. They were all marvellous. I had help all the time. Really, they were very good."

At times I felt excessively tired, and often felt the strong desire to sleep. After I got up, and had begun short excursions down the corridor in the early days of my recovery, I did not like sitting in a chair afterwards, or even on the edge of the bed, because I felt so weary. I simply had to sleep. Terri had much the same experience, even after having been asleep.

> "It's so hard to distinguish whether it's tiredness or the anaesthetic. Your body is using all your energy just to recover and heal itself. All the energy I had was used getting up and going to the toilet, showering, talking to my visitors. Even that became tiresome sometimes if they were coming one after another."

Feelings about recovery

During my recovery I sometimes wondered whether I would ever feel better, and at other times I was elated at the remarkable progress I was making. These cycles of elation and frustration also appeared among my informants. They centred on ideas and feelings about personal dignity, independence, fear, depression, ridding oneself of the 'wrong' mental attitude, struggling to find the 'right' mental attitude, appreciation of changes to one's body, and a sense of personal achievement.

Being reduced to a child-like role in relation to adults is difficult for some people to bear, but no trouble to others. After a serious operation the role is played in a state of extreme tiredness, with nothing in reserve and little to fall back on.

Mario observed that once the pain of the early recovery had gone, and he was beginning to move about, he forgot the problems of being a patient.

> "One aspect is you do forget. At the moment I can't remember. Maybe I don't want to remember, because now the pain's gone, and you just forget so quickly afterwards."

By contrast, Nell remembered the lack of dignity when ill and that illness eroded her sense of modesty while she tried so hard to be independent again.

> "So much indignity. All sense of modesty and dignity has to go out the window, doesn't it? Independence goes, too. But at that stage I think I was quite happy to be dependent on the nurses."

Nell recognised the problems of developing the right mental attitude to the task of being a patient. She remembered that the difficulties were getting through the pain, thinking how long it would last, and forcing yourself to be patient about the recovery.

To feel independent again was what drove Doug.

"They assist you into bed and out of bed. But I learned to hook my right foot underneath the left so that I could support it. I got as good as I could at that so that I became a little independent. Other people used to ring for the nurse every time they wanted to use the toilet. Independence is a very big thing in a hospital. I think the more independent you are, the more the hospital stay's not so bad."

Through the professional eyes of a psychiatrist Ernst observed his fellow patients, and noted that panic, fear, and depression dominated some people in recovery. He concluded that one's mental attitude affected recovery and considered that the attitude was largely under the patients' control.

"I used to go from room to room and socialise with people. I was up and about and they were in bed, so I'd go and visit everyone. What I noticed was that some people were just either frightened, panicked or fearful. I wouldn't say depressed. They were down about it all. I've got no doubt the positive mental approach has a role to play. I'm not saying it's the whole difference at all. Because in fact the guy I shared a room with for my second operation had a very positive mental approach but still had an awful, much slower recovery."

Apart from childbirth, Wendy's only major experience as a patient had been having her tonsils out. She had been a nurse herself and benefited from the experience. For her it was very much business as usual.

"I had only had my tonsils out, and I suppose I didn't feel very apprehensive. I wasn't really concerned about it. I suppose I was so glad to be getting on with it at that stage."

Betty was delighted that she would stand a little taller after her operation.

"After the operation he said he put a shaft in. Not a plate, a shaft, and I was satisfied the damn thing was over. He said, 'I have given you an inch and three-eighths extra on the shaft. I couldn't afford to put in the full two inches.' So I still have three-eighths of an inch [1 cm] discrepancy, which means I have to wear an orthotic. And I have fallen arches. But he did a very big thing for me."

Terri also appreciated her surgeon's efforts to improve her body.

"The surgeon tended to put the incision round the back for me. It was sweet of him. Shorts would cover it."

Helen made an all-round recovery in hospital, and felt that she had achieved something special for herself.

"I felt really, really good in hospital this time. I just felt that I actually had a divine light. I had friends I hadn't seen for a long time coming in. I felt loved and cared for, really wanted, and I felt absolutely brilliant, actually. My skin was really good. After fights over my diet with the kitchen, I managed to get my diet absolutely perfect, and I just felt really good and was looking really good. I hadn't had any intoxicants, any pot [marijuana], I hadn't had any alcohol, I hadn't had anything. I just felt very clear."

Entertainment in hospital

My days were spent watching television well into the night, sleeping, and reading. Although reading was my main occupation, I was not able to concentrate sufficiently on a book to warrant keeping it beside me. I listened to some books on tape. Above the bed was a small television screen; it had several radio stations incorporated in it and could be used with earphones so that the man in the bed beside me was not disturbed. In my hand I had a remote control device that changed channels.

Sonomi was anxious to recover quickly and return to her work, but recognised that recovery would not be as rapid as she wanted. She tolerated the interruptions of normal hospital life and enjoyed her visitors. Even so she fought with herself and fretted a little at the slow rate of recovery.

"I had a lot of visitors and a lot of beautiful flowers too, and telephone calls. I ended up getting back to some work. Sometimes people from my gallery would come in and we'd talk about things. I felt I could do that.

Attention span and interest in really complicated reading is set back quite a bit. I found I was only interested in very short things, things that were easy to glance through. I brought in oodles of books and opened only two of them. There were always noises, and people coming in."

Bernard watched television, picked books up and put them down, and didn't read a lot because to concentrate on reading was an effort. Terri had much the same experience.

"People brought me magazines in hospital. I literally couldn't look at them until a few days before I was due to come home. I always remember my university teacher saying to me once, 'Oh, when you're in hospital you can read and study.' You can't study. In the past, because I read a lot, I've taken books into hospital, but they're a waste of time. You just can't read. It was week and a half before I could even flick through a magazine."

On the other hand, Charles said he read a few books in the first week or so.

Social life in hospital

Each day I was happy to see evening visitors, and sometimes we would have a meal together in the hospital. Friends would call during the day and join me for morning or afternoon tea or coffee. Flowers were delivered. One evening three female friends arrived, one with champagne and glasses. The nurse drew the curtain around me with a slight frown, and nodded in understanding when I claimed not to know the visitors at all well.

In my ward was a friendly accountant who ran his own firm. For at least a week after his operation he was on the phone regularly to his office, and every other evening he had a conference beside his bed with his staff. He never stopped working, or so it seemed, because he was in the middle of a difficult case. He seemed to find recovery slow and painful, and said that when he did recover fully he would again be able to dash across the city street outside his office to catch the tram. After three or four days a single room became vacant and I was told that it was mine. I suggested to the nurse that the accountant take the room because he seemed to need privacy for his business affairs. She agreed.

So for a day or so I was in a double room alone. Later I had two companions. One was an elderly war veteran who had had a hip replaced about ten years ago and had recently fallen in the gravel along his driveway. The pain had spread, and he was advised to have his hip replaced again. The other man was a garrulous and cheerful sportsman with considerable business interests and a wide range of community duties. He talked at length about his activities until he was anaesthetised, operated on for a knee complaint, and sent home.

Other informants were not so fortunate in their fellow patients. After his operation Fred was taken back to his ward and found he was with a fellow patient whom he saw before the operation and had hoped he would never see again. Doug had the same experience and was offered the chance to move, but decided he would stay in the six-bed ward, where he learned much from his fellow patients.

> "The day after the operation I was starting to get back to where I was. They had a shared room available for me, and now I felt obligated to these fellows I had got to know. I wasn't going to walk out on them. So I ended up staying where I was, and that was a good thing. We could discuss things, and each of the fellows was a bit in front of me. Two people had hips done, and two had knees done. I had a good cross-section of patients. I learned what to expect."

On principle Terri did not want to sleep and live in a room with a stranger.

> "I can't stand being in with other people when I'm sick. I don't want their visitors; I just want to be by myself. All my energy is for seeing my own visitors."

Betty was put in a room with someone she did not want to be with, and decided not to use the TV and to feign sleep in the hope that the woman would not try to talk to her.

> "There was this awful woman who had her hip done. She was there on the day I went in, and unfortunately she was in my ward. So I didn't use the television and radio. I just wanted to look as though I was asleep to the lady next door."

Helen did not like being alone. She had a happy time with one fellow patient, but was tempted to violence against another.

"I am a social animal. I had a lovely person who was wonderful. She'd fallen down a manhole that had been left unattended and broken her hip, and then had terrible traumas getting it right again. Occasionally you might get someone you don't like. If you hassle the nurses enough they'll move you. Three years ago I was in with this woman who just whinged and carried on, and I was in' terrible pain. I had visions of murdering her. I told the nurses."

Mario shared with others and, until a less than acceptable new patient arrived, appreciated the company.

"A private room had been offered to me, not immediately, but during the recovery time, and I said I was happy to be in shared accommodation. There were four in the room, three at first, and then this fourth person came in. That was fine because it was company. However, some time into the recovery period there was a new patient who was a problem, a vocal problem. Not just vocal in terms of pain, but an irritating person who wasn't a good patient. I did ask if I could have a private room. Had they had a spare room, I think they would've acceded to the request."

After leaving hospital

Coming home

Before I went into hospital we decided that I would not go to a rehabilitation centre to recover, but that I would be looked after at my home by the sea, which is two hours drive from the hospital. I left hospital with a toilet seat, a pair of elbow crutches, my soap on a rope, an extension arm that a friend had lent me, as well as a small bed rug of sheepskin to go under the sheet to make me comfortable sitting up in bed. I wore the TED/DVT white stockings that I had used in hospital. At the reception desk there was a small sum to be paid to the hospital for long-distance phone calls; otherwise the major expenses were paid to the hospital by my health insurer. I had an appointment to see my surgeon in four weeks.

Doug came home after nine days in hospital, and his wife, who works part-time, was there to look after him. Fred was pleased to leave the hospital after ten days of discomfort and poor nursing. His wife, a former nurse, cared for him. He was on two under-arm crutches. He used a walking frame for about three days after the operation. Charles left to go home with two crutches, a pillow, and a stiff hip. Mario, who did not know that he could have gone to a rehabilitation centre, went home after about ten days. His doctor insisted he go home in an ambulance. After five days in hospital Ernst went home to be looked after by his doctor wife.

Sonomi lives alone, so she arranged for an occupational therapist to come to her home before she attended the pre-admission clinic. She did not want to return home after the operation and not be able to manage. A therapist called a week before she went to hospital, checked her home for no charge, and friends also came to help.

Rehabilitation centres

The role of the rehabilitation centres is changing. In the past it was appropriate for patients to decide for themselves whether to go to a rehabilitation centre before returning home. Some would stay a few days, others two or more weeks. Today the cost of rehabilitation is rising fast. In future some health insurers might not offer this option to their clients, and the choice of a rehabilitation centre or home might not be as readily available as it once was. Changes in the management of recovery from hip replacement operations also indicate that the best practice might be to have the patient cared for at home, if possible, rather than spending time at a rehabilitation centre. For older people, and especially those who have no one at home to care for them, a rehabilitation centre is mandatory. But for people who are young, fit, recovering rapidly in hospital, and have a capable carer at home, home might be the best place for the next two to four weeks. The decision is best made in consultation with your family or other carers and the surgeon after the hip has been replaced.

Sonomi, Nell, and Betty went to a rehabilitation centre before coming home. Each stayed for a different period. Betty was told she could attend the centre for as long as she felt that she needed their help.

"I went every day and I did my exercises, either in the gym or elsewhere. I still do them, every morning. In the rehabilitation centre they gave me tablets, two prescribed painkillers, two sleeping tablets, two bowel opening medicines. It was very routine and disciplined there, which I appreciated very much. They made me wear the long white stockings. They gave them to me to bring home. I just couldn't get those on myself, because the bending was hard, so I did need somebody to help me there.

> They gave me a thing that helps socks to go on. They offered me a chair under the shower, but I happened to have one."

Nell, who was in hospital for thirteen days, spent two weeks in a rehabilitation centre, before going home. She was most appreciative of her time at the rehabilitation centre.

> "I was worried because I had to come home to a tiny flat, which was not easy to get around in, and a bathroom with little space to move in. It was essential to have those two weeks at the rehabilitation place. It set me up, really. That was marvellous. You go more or less at your own pace, and you have hydrotherapy."

Sonomi went to a rehabilitation centre where her general practitioner had arranged her admission. At the centre she was supervised by another doctor whom she rarely saw. Nurses attended to her closely, and she also had the benefit of an occupational therapist and a physiotherapist. On arriving she was assigned to a room overlooking a busy main road, refused to occupy the room, and insisted she have a room with less traffic noise. She was given the room she wanted and settled in for a week. Physiotherapy extended the exercises she had done in bed while in hospital, and they were augmented with standing exercises.

> "I would go once a day to the physio room, do basic exercises, walking, upstairs and downstairs, moving from crutches to sticks as soon as possible."

Occupational therapy focused on the restrictions that would become evident when a patient got home, and because most patients at the rehabilitation centre were elderly, and many were recovering from a stroke, their needs were different from Sonomi's. She was not interested in how to cope in her kitchen while she was temporarily disabled, and felt that, not being elderly, she had no need of advice and practices in the home offered by the occupational therapist.

> "My whole idea was to pick up the 'what-ifs' and the 'how-tos' for when I came back home where I didn't have anyone. It was not structured to help with anything. People like me knew how to cook. What people needed to know was how to bend, how to move things from A to B in a kitchen."

Nevertheless she felt the centre was useful because it offered her help with everyday activities, and consequently the independence that she needed to survive, for example getting dressed with the extension arm, and being guided by the physiotherapist in how much further she could go with her exercises.

Around home

Sitting

Shortly after I got home my daughter arrived with a carver chair with arms. I had a similar modern dining room chair. One was put at each end of a long room. They became my major places to sit. It was not possible to lounge or sit in a low armchair for about two weeks.

Helen was not permitted to use a chair at all for a while.

"At home I wasn't put in a chair. I just wasn't allowed to put any weight on the hip at all. You've got to be fairly careful moving about."

Bedroom

At night I slept on my back, as instructed, with a pillow between my legs. I slept on the left side of the bed with two crutches nearby, so that I could get up in the way I had been shown in hospital. I slept well and stayed in bed until about 10 a.m. each day. This was not the case for Charles, who was unable to sleep when he got home because he had to sleep on his back.

"When I got home I was no better. Dreadful. My general health deteriorated quite dramatically. I've kept in good health, fortunately. But I was, for that period, that winter, very bad. Just wasn't sleeping."

When I got up and dressed I wore cotton slacks that could be pulled on easily, a light shirt, and the white Velcro-tabbed shoes. I needed help putting on the long white TED/DVT stockings, every day for four weeks. Other socks were not necessary. After two weeks I could easily remove the white stockings myself.

When dressing I found the extension arm was invaluable for securing my shoes, and picking up clothes when dressing myself. I did not use a sock aid or the long shoehorn because the shoes opened wide. Ernst found the sock aid very useful and, like most others, found the extension arm most valuable. Charles did not use the extension arm much; his wife put on his socks. But Nell appreciated the extension arm and also used the sock aid.

"I had a plastic extension arm. They're wonderful things. I put my sock on with a thing like cardboard [sock aid]. It was sort of curved. You put it into your sock or tights and then pull the string."

Bathroom

The seat in the toilet was adjusted for my height, 188 cm (6 ft 2 in), and was quite comfortable. I lowered it after two weeks so that I could gradually get used to the regular height of toilet seats. The shower was over the bath, and was not safe. For a few days, I showered outside under a garden shower connected to hot water by hose. At first it was difficult to get the temperature right, but after three or four showers that way I braved the bathroom shower. I was surprised to find I could get in and out of the bath easily, and stand securely on a rubber non-slip mat under the shower. The soap on a rope was within reach.

Doug used the special chair for the toilet but not for long, and stood in the shower recess without a chair.

"I found that I could get down and get up. We hired it for a week, but I used it for only two or three days. No problem showering because we have a separate shower."

Charles found the bathroom hazardous.

"I showered with difficulty in a shower recess which I stepped into with some trepidation. I was very uncertain standing; I didn't like to put any weight on my hip. At the hospital pharmacy I rented a raised toilet seat to take home, set to my height."

Ernst recovered quickly, and put the toilet seat and special chairs aside.

"I didn't need a seat in the shower after the first nine days. I didn't need the toilet booster seat or a high chair after a week."

Helen used a raised toilet seat in the bath shower, but found it hazardous.

"The toilet seat didn't actually fit the shower properly. I had to put it in the bath with its back legs hanging over the edge of the bath. During winter it was a bit uncomfortable, and a bit nasty."

Nell hired a toilet seat and wooden seat to place across her bath. Like Helen, she had a shower over the bath, but invented a clever way to dry her feet.

"You could sit on that seat and have the water coming on you. I managed to get rid of that within a week or so. I used a long plastic ruler, about 15 to 18 inches [40 cm], with a little bit of towelling that I could take off and wash. It slipped on to the end like a sock. And that was for drying in between the toes."

Mario also rented a toilet seat, but all he could recall was the story about the friend who took it back when he had finished with it.

"I asked a friend to return the toilet. I didn't think there was anything strange about asking her to take it. Neither did she. I just thought of it as the thing you'd sit on in the shower. But she had to take it on a tram, and was appalled at other passengers looking at this thing and wondering what it was for! That became a bit of a family joke."

Blood testing and monitoring

I wore the TED/DVT white stockings in hospital and for four weeks afterwards. Not all patients do.

I had been instructed to take prescribed tablets, warfarin, an anticoagulant, to keep my blood thin, and to wear the white stockings. Every two or three days a nurse would come to my home to take a blood sample, stay for a short conversation, and telephone at the end of the day to say how many tablets of what colour to take. She said I should take the tablets at the same time every day. Immediately after her call we set a time for taking the tablets. In a booklet provided by the hospital I kept a record of the tablets taken, and in every other way made a religion of her instructions.

Others followed much the same regimen. Doug reported the same procedure. Charles was a subject in a supervised experiment and had a different experience.

"I didn't have white stockings. I had to self-inject with an anticoagulant. It was in lieu of anticoagulant tablets. In the hospital, they taught me how to do the daily injection in the fleshy part of the stomach. And I did that for four weeks at home."

Betty was familiar with the procedure for preventing blood clots because of her husband's illness. She did not use the stockings, but had an injection in the area near her stomach.

Mario also did not wear the white stockings, and understood the purpose of the tablets.

"I don't know why the white stockings would be used. I had a course of tablets when I came home. I think blood clots was one reason for them."

Ernst had the TED/DVT stockings and saw their change in the brief interval between his two operations.

"I was supposed to have had the stockings for six weeks and the same with the anticoagulants. I stopped both after four weeks, with the surgeon's agreement. He recognised that I was so active. I was going for daily long walks on the crutches. Deep vein thromboses are much more common in people who are resting in bed and not very active. I found the stockings quite inconvenient coming to work, hot and uncomfortable. For the first operation I had to wear the ones that hooked up to a suspender belt. I used to joke about having to get my suspenders on. But for the second operation they changed the management, and my surgeon said studies now are showing that shorter stockings above or below the knee are as effective in preventing deep vein thrombosis as the ones going up to a suspender belt."

Helen never used white stockings and had no blood tests, and guessed it must have been because she was so young.

"I had no white stocking routine, no blood tests. The woman next to me did. I'm glad I didn't have that. She was in her sixties."

Nell recalled having frequent blood samples for blood clotting and taking differently coloured tablets, but she did not wear white stockings. Tess remembered that ten years earlier she didn't have white stockings, but after more recent operations she did.

Exercising

Walking

My recovery routine was established early and followed a predictable and comforting pattern. In time I became less and less weary, walked further each day, and gradually re-established my independence. The main adventure was a ten-minute walk from home along the golf links road to a point overlooking the beach. I made it the first challenge. It took two days before I felt I could do that easily.

Charles had a very much slower recovery at home.

"I walked round the house for a start. Then I got out on the street. I just increased it gradually. It was six months before I felt steady. Then I got back on the bike."

Mario followed a routine given by the hospital, while Bernard planned challenging walks around the small seaside town where he lived.

"Now I can go around the block to the post office and back. I do that every morning. I have another route down the back lane. It's a little bit rough. I prefer the flat ground on a good surface."

Doug did much the same, walked a little further each day, rid himself of the crutches, and used a walking stick. But his self-directed recovery was too quick, and he had to return to crutches for a week after he went back to work.

Ernst recovered much faster than others and, like Doug, had to be restrained by his surgeon.

"Less than three days after the first operation I walked 800 metres [half a mile] with my crutches. They didn't tell me I wasn't allowed to leave the hospital, so I just got the crutches and walked down the street and back. I had no problem, no pain, no nothing. I went back for the six-week check-up. I hadn't been told that I had to use crutches all the time, and after four weeks I got sick of them. I'd thrown away one crutch after two weeks, and the second one after four weeks. My surgeon said, 'Where are your crutches?' And I said, 'Well, I was walking fine, I thought I didn't need them.' Even so he put me back on one crutch for two weeks."

After his second operation Ernst established for himself what his surgeon expected and held to his instructions.

Terri had a surgeon who cared little for physiotherapy in her case. She was to do her daily tasks, more each day, and to use two sticks. So she took charge of her own recovery at home without doing special exercises.

"My surgeon said if you can walk, just start achieving more everyday tasks. Don't let your leg cross the line down the middle of your body. Do not put your sock on before six weeks. I was not supposed to bend down. I was very well informed on what you can or can't do. I can kneel, but it's very difficult because of the arthritis in my knees. Coming up to six weeks I was well and truly able to start using one stick. And he said, 'I want to see you six weeks after that. If you're at the stage where you feel you can use no stick for a few steps here and there, then do it.' So it's three months before I completely got off a walking aid."

She tackled a flat lane at the back of her house a day or so after getting home. And like Ernst she took things into her own hands and overdid the walking.

"I walked half way and then back, and then I was fine. The next day I walked the whole length, and I was exhausted for three days."

Betty also enjoyed the achievement of recovery but, like others who recover too fast, did not impress the specialist she saw for blood pressure problems.

"I came out of hospital with two sticks, and then I got down to one stick. It's a terrific achievement when you go off two sticks on to one stick, and then no stick. I went to my specialist, and said to her, 'Look, I don't have a stick!' She knew all about the hip operation because she's interested in my health generally, and she said, 'I prefer all my old patients to use a stick.' I felt so flattened. So I've still got a stick."

Walking became Helen's favourite pastime, wherever she was. She used underarm crutches.

"I've always had a limp. They never seem to get the legs the right length. I can walk, you know. I've walked all over Papua New Guinea, I've walked all over Indonesia. I've done an enormous amount of bushwalking."

Nell used crutches for a couple of weeks at home, and then used sticks for a short period. She was afraid to let the elbow crutches go. Her surgeon advised her to put them down when she felt secure.

> "These paths here are very uneven, and I hung on to that stick for quite a long time. I just can't remember how long. Probably longer than necessary."

About three weeks after coming home, I was able to walk the kilometre to the local store and get the newspaper myself. I shall never forget the day I stood outside the store, steadied myself for the steps into the shop, walked in, and the woman at the counter said: 'Look, no crutches!' I smiled, and shrugged happily. I was able to walk without discomfort and to be independent. There was only a week to go before I had to see the surgeon to get the all-clear and drive the car again. Then it was off to work. That last week of recovery was one of the best vacations I can remember.

Hydrotherapy

I did not undergo hydrotherapy myself, but I visited a hydrotherapy pool to observe what the physiotherapist did for her patients. Patients who have heart problems or skin problems are checked for them before they are allowed to go into the pool.

If your wound has healed properly you are ready for hydrotherapy. Usually this is between four and six weeks after the operation, except when you go to a rehabilitation centre, where you might take hydrotherapy well before that because you are in a closely supervised and well-protected environment. Some patients would go in at the two-week mark.

Hydrotherapy involves moving in water using the resistance of the water to help strengthen muscles. Sessions last about a half an hour. The pool is comfortable and warm. In a rehabilitation centre patients do hydrotherapy every day. If you are not in such a centre, you would go three or four times a week.

Many items are used to help you float; some you lie on, others are tied around your feet, others you hold in your hands. Exercises include walking in the water forwards, backwards, and sideways. Each direction uses different muscles. You can march underwater, pick up your knees, swing the leg sideways, and stand on one foot and squat. You can swim to the corner of the pool, and, with your back to the corner, hold on to the rail at water level, cycle your legs under water, spread them apart, bring them together, and kick with legs straight.

Some people have problems with hydrotherapy, but they are easily managed. If you do not float securely, special floats are tied around you to keep you close to the surface. The warmth of the water diminishes feelings of pain. It gives some people a false sense of well-being and leads them to overdo their exercises. When they emerge from the pool, they suddenly feel heavy and begin to hurt. Consequently, hydrotherapy is closely supervised by a physiotherapist.

In the first session patients are shown basic exercises, which many do for two or three weeks; when they come back, they are given more advanced exercises. You need to be confident to do the advanced exercises. An advanced activity would be to take a board and go paddling up and down the length of the pool, as swimmers in training do. Older people who do not like to lie back in the water and get their hair wet can do standing exercises.

The therapist follows a principle that exercise must advance exertion but not to the point of pain. The therapist advances the effort needed to do the exercises by putting a slightly greater strain on the patient at each session and leading the patient gently to the next level of exertion.

Hydrotherapy is valuable to patients because it lets them share their treatment process with others, and helps them learn what to expect when they progress to the next stage of their therapy.

Doug found that hydrotherapy helped him to regain his confidence about walking.

"As soon as I left the hospital, when my cut was healed enough, I went to do hydrotherapy at the local pool. I found it the best thing. You can get in there without a walking stick. You can't fall over. I went for an hour every day. I happened to know one of the physios down there, and she showed me a number of things to do. Not just walking up and down in the water, but also side-stepping in the water and walking backwards in the water. And the other one was swinging your leg to the side, the middle, then up. Progressively you swing it a little bit higher and wider. It gave me confidence."

It is cheaper for you do the exercises yourself after one or two sessions, because each time you see the physiotherapist you pay a fee. Fees might be claimable on your medical insurance.

At her rehabilitation centre Nell enjoyed the hydrotherapy.

"I did all sorts of things around the edge and across the pool. There were lots of exercises like ballet steps and marching, lifting the legs. That wasn't easy, either."

Even though Sonomi did not enjoy spending time in water, she found hydrotherapy at her rehabilitation centre most valuable in helping her to strengthen her operated leg.

"The water's terribly warm. You can whip around in the water without any help at all. I don't like water, but I went every day. I could see that I could do things. That was helpful."

Exercise routines

My surgeon recommended that I walk as far as possible each day. I had plans to travel overseas for a conference in six weeks; he seemed to think it would be all right.

I did the bedroom exercises and walked; nothing else. I did not know how long the convalescence would take. Others took a more active interest in extending their exercise program. When Charles came home he adopted the vigorous attitude shown by his physiotherapist in hospital.

"When I came home I would be exercising three times a day for thirty-five minutes, then I increased the number of movements at about eight or ten weeks after the operation. I kept doing them for three months. I was resigned to a long convalescence, and I had largely stripped my commitments to accommodate it, so I wasn't worried."

After six weeks of exercises, he began to swim.

Bernard felt that he wanted some new exercises and went to his local chiropractor, who gave him an exercise not on the list from hospital.

"You lie on your side with the pillow between your legs, and lift them. First couple of times I thought, 'Oh, my God, I'm not going to be able to do this.' But now I can lift my legs a couple of times."

Nell went to a rehabilitation centre where the exercise program was more elaborate than what she had been shown in hospital.

"There were lots of exercises. A bicycle with the pedals was attached to the wall. You sit there, they adjust the seat, and you try and get around. That was difficult even to start with. It was amazing that you couldn't get right round at first. But eventually you'd get right round."

Car travel

I had to sit in the front seat, and did not drive until my surgeon said so. You will not be able to sit in a rear seat because your operated leg would be beyond the 90-degree limit.

Before you get into the car on the passenger's side, have the seat pushed back as far as it will go, and tilt it back a little. Back yourself into the car as far as the seat will allow, and then turn your back towards the inclined seat. Your operated leg should be as straight as possible. When you have turned you will not find it difficult to place your two feet on the floor in front of you.

I followed the instructions above. On the front passenger seat I put a small pillow in a plastic shopping bag. In position the small pillow made the seat level with the ground rather than sloping downwards towards the upright back of the seat. I backed into the front seat, and on to the pillow. Because the pillow was slippery in its plastic bag, I could turn easily to face the front of the car. My operated leg was strong enough to lift itself into the footwell. There was no discomfort during my two-hour journey home from hospital.

I was not permitted to drive a car until five weeks after I was discharged from hospital. Had the car been an a automatic, perhaps it would have been four weeks. It seemed much longer for Betty.

"I have an automatic car, which should have been all right because it was the left hip, but I couldn't drive the car for probably three or more months."

Because he was so athletic, Ernst was driving himself much sooner after the operation.

"After a week and a half I was driving again. I've got an automatic because I couldn't change gears for the last five years with my left leg."

Terri drove an automatic too, and returned to driving after six weeks.

Charles, Doug and Nell had a new hip in their right leg. Each informant had quite different experiences. Charles was at home for almost twelve weeks.

"I didn't get out of the house because I was told not to get in the car and drive for three months. The right leg would be on the accelerator."

Doug relied on what it felt like to use the brake in his car.

"Having the right leg done was a restriction. You do everything with it in an automatic car, and you wouldn't have the same problems if you'd had your left hip done. The left hip does very little in a modern automatic car. So it was only a matter of feeling that I could push with some authority on the brake pedal."

Nell was more concerned about getting in and out of the car than driving it.

"I was desperate about driving a car, and waited about six weeks. I drive an automatic, and the operation was on my right hip. It took me a while to get in and out of the car easily. I did it slowly."

Entertainment

To entertain myself while recovering at home I read a few books, listened to the radio and books on tape, read magazines and newspapers, enjoyed breakfast in bed, wrote cards to people who had visited me in hospital, and at night sat before the fire and watched television. Each weekend I had dinner or lunch with visitors who came to witness the stages of my recovery, talk about the people they knew who had also had their hips done, and lighten the burden of secluded life. In this way the four weeks raced by.

Doug too was happy to sit at home, read a book, and wait for the nurse to come and test his blood. But for Terri the transition from hospital to home was not easy. She felt ambivalent towards what she would do at home.

"When I came home, I had more things to do. At home your energy goes, and you still don't want to read. I just lay on the couch and watched television. I actually don't adjust well to coming home. I hate coming home, yet I want to get home. It's a very hard transition for me."

Sex life

Before getting new hips, many people have difficulty enjoying sex because of pain and stiffness, especially in the hips and knees. Also, your partner might have avoided sex for fear of causing you further discomfort or pain.

With your new hip you might find that your joint pain and stiffness are gone, and you might want to start having sex again. There is no medical reason to suppose that your sex life is incompatible with having a new hip. About four to six weeks is the average time people wait before resuming sexual activity. Your wound has healed, and muscles and ligaments are recovering well by this time.

The questions you might ask are: are you physically and emotionally ready? Do you understand clearly the care you should take to safeguard your new hip? The first question is answered with little difficulty if, during the waiting period, however long, you keep sharing non-sexual acts of intimacy, physical and verbal, and keep physically close, touch, hold hands, hug, and kiss as a matter of course.

The second question is answered best with a few precautions. Initially there might be some pain when you start having sex again. Talk about the pain or discomfort, as you would any intimate matter with the person you love. Regard it as an experiment in which you are finding the best way to return to a gratifying sex life. Your partner might feel rejected and frustrated, and wonder if he or she is hurting you. Talking and laughing about the hazards of being a sex athlete with a new hip might clear away the uncertainties and ambivalence of taking up where you had to leave off.

The first precaution concerns how you do it. For three months, or until your surgeon says otherwise, to reduce stress on the new hip, you must be careful, if lying on your back, to avoid raising the operated leg beyond the 90-degree point, and try not to let your operated leg roll towards the other leg.

If you lie on your side, the non-operated side, keep the affected leg outside the midline of your body, that is, try not to cross your operated leg over the other.

The second precaution concerns where you do it. You will find it is best for you to take the bottom position at first. In this position keep the operated leg to the side, toes pointing to ceiling. To support your affected leg, and to feel comfortable, a bed pillow can be put under your affected thigh. Don't bend your hip, and do not be too vigorous.

Men and women can also lie on the side. If you are a woman, roll on your unaffected side and place two — maybe more — pillows between your legs to keep your hip in a safe position; again, do not bend the hip more than 90 degrees. The pillows should be in a position that supports your operated leg and stops it from rolling off the pillows while becoming active.

If you are a man, roll on to you unaffected side and use your partner's legs to support the affected leg. While active you should keep your affected leg on top of your partner's leg. Meanwhile your partner should have at least two pillows between her legs to help keep your hip in a safe position. Again, the 90-degree rule should be observed.

For men both the top position and the sitting position are appropriate.

In the top position remember not to twist or turn your operated leg towards the other leg when rolling yourself from your back to your stomach. Keep the operated leg to the side, toes pointed outward. As always, observe the 90-degree rule.

To enjoy the pleasure and intimacy of sex after you have a new hip, you will need to be have a positive mental attitude to sex, the ability to laugh a little at the newness of it all, and an experimental view of sex with your new hip. If at first things do not seem right, explore other ways of having sex, and remember: with a little practice you will be as good as ever you were.

Only one of my informants volunteered comments about sex. The person said that within six weeks a gratifying sex life had returned for both patient and partner.

"I enjoy a good sex life, and I was finding that I was really inhibited, I couldn't extend the hips, and it was a real problem. But since I've had the operation, I have been able to have intercourse normally. Much sooner than the book was saying."

Your surgeon is the person to see if you find that having sex is painful.

Sport

Your new hip is designed for walking, using stairs, and sedentary activities. For walking thick cushioned soles are recommended. When you carry a suitcase or groceries, lift no more than 12 kg (25 lb). The same goes for a small backpack when hiking. When you carry weighty items be sure they are lifted on the same side as your operated leg.

Most surgeons recommend that you turn to the gentle sports, with no body contact, no jarring or impacting of the hip, no sudden lurching, twisting and turning. Bowls, a quiet game of tennis, a round of golf, riding a stationary bike, non-weight-bearing callisthenics, and plenty of walking are strongly recommended. A quiet game of tennis means keeping your knees bent and moving with the good foot. Playing doubles is preferred. Some surgeons would not recommend horse riding or skiing. If you are an athlete, gentle hip-girdle exercises four times a week would be appropriate. Hiking with a light pack might be allowed. Little support is given to fishing in a stony stream, jogging, running a long distance, lifting weights, treadmill training, squash, baseball, basketball, volleyball, football of any kind, cross-country skiing, ice-skating, hockey, or cricket. Skiing is frowned upon, but I have heard of some people who ski well with a new hip. Parachuting is not a good idea, nor is deep-sea fishing or scuba diving.

About ten months after my operation I played a round of golf with one friend who had had a new hip about two years previously. He walked normally and did not get tired. I did. Thereafter I went to a driving range to maintain the skill of hitting the ball, and each day I walked as far as I could, about 5 km (3 miles). A year after the operation, I was ready to resume golf.

My surgeon was quite definite about what I was allowed to do: no jumping, jogging, tennis, or skiing. For me, swimming replaced jogging. I was permitted to do anything else, for example, kneeling and stretching, but I was not to cross my legs in such a way that my left knee was raised close to my right hip. It is in this position that the left hip (the operated hip in my case) can dislocate, and this is the reason for the golden rule: do not sit with your legs crossed. He showed me that it was all right to put the left ankle on the right knee while sitting.

Helen is not able to run. Her exercise is swimming.

"I don't play contact sport because I'm not allowed to, and I wouldn't want to. I've always been a good swimmer; I don't do as much as I probably should."

Ernst, a devoted sportsman, was advised by his surgeon to play golf, a new sport for him.

"I'm a hopeless golfer. Two weeks after the operation I started practising golf, no problems. I'm playing at a par 3 course until I learn how to play. I'm improving, and I'm doing a lot of practice, of course. Actually I played eighteen holes of golf just six days after my gall bladder was out."

Returning to work

I returned to my office eight weeks after the operation. I travelled to work in crowded trains, buses, and trams because I was not permitted to drive my manual car. It was a new experience to find people standing aside for me, and several times I was offered seats in the crowded compartments of trains and near the entrance of trams.

Nell worked part-time, was away for two months, and found that driving her car rather than working itself raised problems for her.

"I took the stick to work with me to start with, just to feel sure when I was getting in and out of the car, and that sort of thing."

Ernst was aware that patients are advised to be away from work for six weeks, and knew that even that duration is not enough for some. He decided that three weeks would be enough for him. He went back to work because of an emergency after two weeks. In his consulting rooms he carefully organised his seating because much of his time is spent listening to patients. Again, it is clear that if you are physically fit, recovery can be remarkably rapid.

"Before returning to work I had organised a special high chair to sit in. I found that, a week after the operation, I could sit in low chairs without any problems at all, and for the first six weeks I was still trying not to go more than 90 degrees. I was careful for the first six weeks. My surgeon said that most dislocations occur in the first six weeks if they're going to occur at all."

8

Problems or complications

At home things will gradually settle back to normal. The hip pain will have diminished, but you will feel uncomfortable, probably for several weeks. Some people have swollen ankles, feel pains in the knee, around the hip, and in the thigh and calf, and worry about their recovery.

After a week at home Sonomi was fretting about her progress. In places her leg felt a little hard and swollen. Was this normal? she asked herself. When will my recovery be complete? How soon will I be fit to work? She had plenty of sick leave, but felt she would much rather be at work than at home. She was frustrated by the waiting. Because she wanted to recover without any mishaps, she became very cautious about the way she stood, turned, and did her exercises. Even so, was she progressing?

Helen felt happy with her recovery in hospital, but when she came home life was not what she anticipated.

"I felt very clear, and spiritually clear in a weird sort of way. And then when I got home it sort of crashed. Once my friend had gone, I was virtually by myself, and it was raining and cold all the time. Then I needed some comfort."

Terri felt weary. No matter how much she rested, the tiredness pervaded all she did.

"No matter how much rest I had, it did not shake that tired feeling. It is something that will just wear off as you recover. I hate that feeling. Before

I came home I felt as if I actually wanted to be here. When I was at home, for at least two weeks it felt as if half of me was still back in that hospital."

Some surgeons simply tell their patients to expect an irregular recovery, insist that they wear the TED/DVT white stockings for four weeks, and that a nurse will come every few days to sample blood and recommend how much warfarin to take.

To make this period more difficult you might drop into old habits, like taking risks by sitting in too low a chair, twisting suddenly, bending or stooping too quickly. To avoid mishaps you are expected to do things slowly, like Sonomi, give thought to your next action, and to keep the spectre of dislocation before you.

Six weeks after the operation I saw the surgeon. I was using a walking stick and felt happy with my recovery. I had gone through all the bumpy moments and frustration about not progressing at a regular pace. I knew that I had a cementless hip, but not what that meant for my recovery rate. I felt frustrated when the surgeon said I was not to drive for a week beyond the period I had been led to believe was appropriate.

My only personal complaint was a feeling of lethargy, especially at night, and a lack of alertness. I thought this was due largely to the after effects of the general anaesthetic. Later I discovered that problems and complications can arise at home during the recovery and for months afterwards, but with time they become less and less likely.

Pain

Your pain is expected to go away after surgery and residual discomfort to diminish gradually. If this is not the case, and pain actually becomes worse, no matter what you do, you are expected to contact your surgeon. Pain might arise in the knee, calf, thigh, or chest or around the wound.

Pain in the knee might be due to arthritis, because the knee carries your weight. Such pain could arise because of the vigorous twisting and turning of your leg during the operation. Knees can take weeks to recover, but eventually they settle and the discomfort goes. If there is pain in the calf associated with tenderness and swelling, you can raise your leg when sitting. The swelling will probably go. But if the swelling increases, becomes too great to ignore, and does not respond to elevation, your surgeon should be told.

Pain in the hip also fades as the wound heals and as the muscles and ligaments repair. If the pain increases steadily, your surgeon should know.

Pain can establish itself in the thigh. I felt such twinges, and even a year later a slight discomfort comes and goes, especially after a heavy day in the garden. The discomfort is so minor that I ignore it. Two years after surgery, I can expect occasional twinges, as the cementless implant secures its place at the points of bone ingrowth. Had it been cemented, such twinges might not have appeared. People with cemented prostheses feel twinges for only brief periods.

Persistent pain in the thigh is found in 10 per cent of people who are given a cementless prosthesis like mine. It is probably due to the readjustments of weight and physical pressures on the bone.

If the pain is severe, the cementless hip might be removed and replaced with a cemented hip. In some cases the cementless hip has been so well encased in bone that to remove the prosthesis might be inappropriate. Tess had this experience.

Pain in the chest can be very serious. If you hurt when you cough or get short of breath, it could be a sign of an **embolism**, and you are expected to tell the surgeon immediately.

After a week at home Fred felt a great pain in his lower back on the left side, opposite the operated hip. He thought that it was due to a strain because he had moved too quickly in bed, and, with rest, in time it would go. But the chest pain persisted. When he phoned the surgeon, Fred was immediately sent to hospital. A blood clot in his legs had broken off and travelled via the veins to his lung. A large clot can reduce the blood supply to the lungs and bring on death. He was treated with blood thinner to stop the clot getting any larger, and he became most anxious about the clot reaching his heart and lungs. He sought advice on how it would be treated, but felt the advice was not clear and the treatment haphazard. He became more anxious. Nevertheless, the treatment proved effective. These days such a complication is rare, but it was probably the major experience that contributed to Fred never wishing to have any more surgery.

This reminds us that death related to getting a new hip is very rare. Nevertheless, it is a known risk.

Pain and infection

Pain in the wound or the area around it can occur because of infection. This is also rare. Some doctors recommend that if you are a long way from medical assistance you should take your temperature twice a day for two months. If it goes above normal, take it three times a day. If you get two abnormally high readings, at least three hours apart, tell the surgeon.

Infection can be superficial or deep. If superficial, the wound feels hot, looks red, and is treatable with antibiotics. If the problem runs deep, it is serious because it centres on the new hip, is not easy to treat, and could require a long period of antibiotics. In some cases the antibiotics might not work. The worst outcome would be to have the new hip replaced.

Infection can be established in many ways. It can arise from the patient's skin or the air in the operating theatre, or it could be spread by blood. It can settle at the site of the prosthesis. Furthermore, the deep infection might not appear for some years after the operation.

To curb the chances of deep infection, modern surgery has effectively used antibiotics during and immediately after the operation. Consequently the chances of this severe complication have been reduced to between 1 and 3 per cent today. It is worth noting that some surgeons do not distinguish between deep and surface infections; to them any infection is a very serious matter.

The possibility of infection is always there. If you have dental work done, a severe sore or infection, or a bad cut that is slow to heal, antibiotics should probably be used. Your doctor and dentist should be told about your new hip.

Sudden changes to the body

Other rare risks that might occur when you get home concern the failure of the body to cope with the shock of having an operation. For example, the kidneys might fail, a very rare occurrence, or, slightly more common but still very unusual, uric acid might build up in the blood so that gout ensues. It can be treated quickly by your doctor.

Terri, who suffers from rheumatoid arthritis, was walking on one stick through shopping centres for up to three hours on some days. She was amazed how quickly her pain had gone. Then her rheumatoid arthritis flared up in all joints.

"Everything was hurting, everything was getting swollen, even finger joints that hadn't been swollen in years."

She believed that this was a common complaint after major surgery and went to see what could be done. After discussions with her doctor she changed her diet radically, rested, and began to accept the complaint.

"We played around with the drugs that I was on, no processed foods, no dairy foods, no meat, and I started eating fish for the first time. I was very immobile. I could do a few things a day, and then I'd be wiped out for the rest of the day. Even now vacuuming can be a bit hard."

Her surgeon indicated that if the distress did not diminish in twelve months she would just have to learn to live with it.

"There's always good and bad with everything. I didn't go in with it. I came out with it. As it happens, I went abroad recently, and I never noticed it when I was over there."

The fluctuations in her discomfort will probably be life-long problems because, although rheumatoid arthritis can resolve spontaneously, arthritis is usually relapsing and remitting or eventually progressive.

Ossification

In the soft tissues around the hip there is a 7 per cent risk of bone emerging in different spots and showing up on the X-ray well after the operation. This is known as ectopic or heterotopic ossification. As a rule the patient is not at any disadvantage. But it might spread and limit movement, especially if it reaches the gap between the femur and the acetabulum. Among those affected, very few find their movement restricted.

Charles was affected this way when a spur of bone appeared about five weeks after the operation. One successful treatment is to have an operation to cut off the spur, then have radiation to the hip. This prospect did not please Charles because of the fear of infection from the hospital.

> "In the sixth week I went to the physiotherapist. She detected that I was not able to raise the leg. The surgeon put me on a course of anti-inflammatories to arrest what was happening. You can see it on the X-ray. There's a spur of bone sticking out. He can go in and take that out, but then you put yourself in the hands of all those golden staph running around inside."

Ernst, too, was concerned that he might have had ossification. To reduce the chance of it establishing itself, he took anti-inflammatory tablets.

Mario had some unusual ossification. He found it worrying because of the sound it made as it healed.

> "When I lay on my operated side I felt an irritation not just under the skin but from the bone. It appears that a spur had grown from the joint that had been cut and had to wear itself out by movement of the muscle. It was a sort of sawing or cutting sound. The pain went away after some time."

Swelling, bruising, bleeding

For a few weeks your ankles might swell. Your surgeon will advise you to elevate the foot when you are not walking. Excessive swelling could be due to blood clots in the veins of the leg. If the swelling is associated with pain and tenderness, or seems excessive and does not go away when you elevate it, you should speak with your surgeon. As a rule, such minor swelling goes within three months.

After surgery you might bleed around the wound, a problem that had worried Doug and was promptly dealt with at the hospital. Some time well after he went home, Mario found a large bruise on his bottom.

"It was the size of a spread hand. I rang the surgeon, and I was assured that it was OK."

It had been caused by the operation and would pass.

In his second hip operation Ernst experienced swelling. He had a drain tube, but it drained little fluid away, and he suffered more swelling than expected.

"I'm sure it was the swelling into the wound that caused more pain over the week or two later. It still wasn't bad, but it was more than the time before."

Long leg illusion

The operated leg might feel too long for the first few weeks, even when the legs are of equal length. For some people this feeling does not go for several months, and they are certain that they will limp forever. There were times when people at work asked me why I was still limping. Others would remark on my gait, saying that I must be better because I was ambling along as I used to. I did not notice this until my attention was drawn to it.

Doug and Betty found that their operated legs were a little longer. Because they had had a lifetime with one leg shorter than the other and limped, getting legs of much the same length was a great bonus.

Accurate measurement during surgery is difficult, and much skill and effort is put into making your legs the same length. It is acceptable to be out a little less than a centimetre (about $1/4$ in). Most people adjust to this difference without noticing. Some patients feel they have legs of different lengths when in fact they are the same.

Why such an illusion? The distance from pelvis to ankle is the *true* length of your leg; the distance from navel to ankle is the *perceived* length of your leg. Most of us experience the perceived and the true length to be the same. But if tight ligaments pull your hip outwards, then your leg will feel too long, even though it is not; consequently, the perceived length of your leg will be *greater* than its true length. If your hip is pulled inwards, it will feel too short, although it is not; in this case, the perceived length of your leg will be *less* than its true length. To solve the problem, be patient, and the illusion will disappear, although your legs will not change in length!

The risk of a real difference in the length of our legs is very slim, about six in a hundred. If one leg is longer than the other, it will be the operated leg. This very rare occurrence raises no problems for mobility, except when nerve damage has occurred. But it does not look right, so it is usually corrected with an orthotic in the shoe, as was the case with Betty.

If ever you need to replace the new hip itself, there is a chance that the first hip will have left you standing a little oddly. You should ask your surgeon whether you can have that corrected so as to regain your original stature. The surgeon cannot guarantee to do so, and might have to lengthen the leg to be sure that you are stable when you recover. Usually the surgeon is faced with a choice between a slightly long leg or a regularly dislocating hip. In this case you will have to be satisfied with a leg that is, in fact, a bit too long.

Walking problems and coordination

When he got home Mario did not feel restricted in what he could do, and expected to recover at a gradual rate. But he did find walking on stairs awkward.

> "I'm pretty well coordinated. Automatically I lead with a certain foot. But I had trouble working out which foot to use, and the only reason I can think of is that I've been used to leading with the other foot."

The most common recommendation for using stairs is an aphorism: put the good leg to heaven, and the bad (operated leg) to hell; in other words, the good leg goes first upstairs, and the bad leg goes first downstairs. With practice this guide provides the necessary habit.

I made two mistakes walking while I recovered. One evening I was out walking and had to step over a small ditch. It was not wide, and I had already stepped over it an hour earlier. I recalled the instructions about walking up stairs. I put the operated leg across the ditch first because the ground was lower on the other side. This was a mistake because suddenly all my weight was on the operated leg. It hurt! Not badly, but it hurt. I did not have my crutches. I walked home gingerly and felt uncomfortable for a day or so.

Several months after the operation, I was getting wood for the fire. It had been raining, and I was wearing some tennis shoes. The ground was wet and a little slippery. Holding two large pieces of wood, I fell on to my right side. It was slow fall and did not hurt, but it gave me a fright. I have not fallen since, and take care to see that I do not.

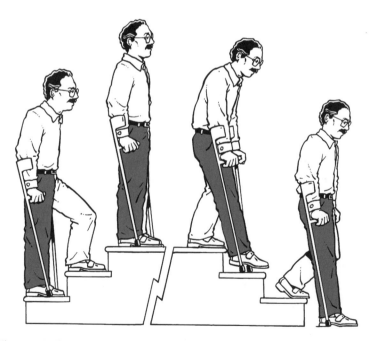

Figure 10: On stairs, step up with the good leg first, and step down with the operated leg first. 'Good leg to heaven; bad leg to hell.'

From time to time I carry a little too much when I empty the car. So I now make an extra trip. My joint will wear, and it will do so sooner the heavier the weight I put on it.

Dislocation

Dislocation is not common and is more likely to happen in the first ten to twelve weeks after surgery. It is difficult to rectify, and is best prevented by using a pillow in bed, a high chair with arms, and a high toilet seat, observing the 90-degree rule, not crossing one's legs or bending suddenly, and exercising regularly to strengthen the leg.

Dislocation of the hip occurs usually with a clunking sound; it is followed by increasing pain. You will be unable to turn your hip or move without added pain. Rarely can a hip dislocate without the person feeling pain. The hip can be put back into place under an X-ray screen with traction or by some special manipulative technique. An anaesthetic could be used, depending on the amount of pain and the procedure employed. Treatment can be followed by a short period of rest in bed, followed by normal walking, which is done with care not to dislocate again.

Ernst, well aware that surgeons are very fearful of dislocations, especially in that first six weeks, heard a click that he thought might indicate dislocation.

"My surgeon, perhaps knowing how physically active I am, never put limits on me. The one thing I did have was what I call 'clicking', and I still get it. The surgeon thinks it's just one of the muscle fascias, the firm parts of the muscle getting on to the prosthesis and then flicking over it. The clicking still happens, but it's not a problem."

Among my informants, none suffered a dislocation.

What else can go wrong?

In an effort to be independent and achieve good health, you can set goals that are too high. Also, failing to accept that you are growing older takes its inevitable toll.

My first challenge was to walk to a special point overlooking the beach. My next challenge was to walk beyond that point, down a hill on the edge of the golf course, and up the hill to home. It was easy. Nevertheless, I spent all the next day in bed. It had been far too strenuous an exercise, and a foolish decision. Without knowing it, I had reached the limits of the recovery process and would have to wait a few days before tackling that challenge again. I settled for my walk to the special point again. A few days later I decided to walk without my elbow crutch. It was a struggle to the point at first. So I took the elbow crutch with me for the second walk that day, but did not use it until I was halfway home. Emboldened by this achievement, I put aside the elbow crutch the following day and would not use it again. That was another mistake. Had I used it for a few more days, I might not have limped about for so long.

High ambition has no place in hip replacement recovery. Neither does showing off. Tess told a story of her great achievement, and how her surgeon tried not to be too impressed.

> "After the first operation I had to go back to my surgeon in six weeks. I went in on one stick. But from the waiting room across to his desk I walked with the stick held up in front of me, and he muttered, 'You're showing off!' It felt that good. That was February. In September we went north and looked after two grandchildren. I was very well."

She had revision surgery because the cement in her new hip had cracked. The second prosthesis was cementless. But in a few years she had hip trouble again and, after a third operation, finds her hip now does not take her weight. She cannot raise her leg on to a step.

> "I've got to drag it up. It just won't take my weight. On the flat, I'm fine. Downhill, I'm fine. But I find climbing steps very difficult. My surgeon doesn't know why because in every X-ray it's been in a perfect position. I had the occasional physiotherapy session for a short time. I don't think I need it. I'm not in pain all the time. My surgeon said, 'No muscle wastage.' He can do everything with my leg. Up, down, round, turn the ankle. Nothing hurts at all, except putting weight on it."

She is restricted in her gardening because she has to hold something to keep her balance when she puts her operated leg forward.

"When I put it forward to pick something up, I find I can't get it back. I can do any high gardening, cutting roses and things, but if I want to do something down low, I am restricted."

She uses an elbow crutch, and keeps one in the car and one in the house. She finds that, several years after the operation, she is very stiff each morning.

"When I've got to go down the driveway for deliveries and other things I use the stick so that I'm not putting too much pressure on this leg to begin with. But during the day the stiffness wears off anyway. I think that's old age, too."

Visiting the surgeon later

I visited the surgeon six and twelve months after the operation. Between the two visits I felt that my recovery was slowing down, that I was hesitating before taking a step when I got out of bed, wondering if my weight was too much for the leg, feeling weary and in need of sleep at unexpected times. I felt my movement was limited, and that I could not kneel comfortably. I could cross my legs easily, and often found myself uncrossing them quickly. After a year the surgeon seemed satisfied that the operation had been a success, but said I should visit him in twelve months.

Doug reported that his surgeon had few questions to ask about his progress and seemed pleased with what had been achieved. Charles's surgeon seemed overjoyed.

"He couldn't stop praising himself! The cement had all become part of the bone, and it'll never wear out. The worst that can happen will be that the head will wear out, but I'll never have cracking. Because apparently these things break down. Cracks in the cement, crumbling cement. You get infection, and it affects your legs, and it's a terrible job to get the thing out. He assures me now that mine is in such good position it will never dislodge."

Ernst's surgeon said that he had put in a good hip.

"So good that if I find I can do more than 90 degrees, he said go for it. I might sound as if I'm a bit cavalier, but all went ahead of schedule.

Except that I made a mistake ditching the crutches too early. I've got an advantage, having some medical knowledge, and the surgeon being a personal friend. I can raise my leg to 90 degrees all the time. I go higher than that. I don't limit it. I've got so much mobility! Once I couldn't do up my own shoelaces except with extreme difficulty, and now I can, no problem at all. It's fantastic."

Betty had made her surgeon happy, too.

"Every year he looks at the X-rays and says, 'Perfect, perfect', and he's quite elated at the condition. I don't know if it's just an ordinary hip operation or because of the extra bit he added to my height. But he's more than satisfied. I'm happy with it."

From a surgeon's point of view there is much more to a successful operation than a good set of X-rays. Watching, observing, and listening to the patient regularly are vital to the surgeon's assessment of the work done and the possibility of complications.

Complications in the long term

Six months or more after the operation complications can occur. Friction of the new hip can create tiny pieces of debris, which loosen the new hip and establish inflammation and some bone loss. This condition, called **osteolysis**, is detected in the X-rays that your surgeon takes at regular intervals after the operation. The loosening has been found in between 30 and 45 per cent of patients ten years after the operation.

With such loosening, bone can gradually disappear. Also there is a slim chance that if your bone strength generally decreases, fractures can occur near the top of the femur. They can heal themselves, but sometimes revision surgery is called for and bone grafts are needed.

These days a very rare complication is the fracturing of part of the prosthesis itself, and this makes revision surgery troublesome.

Six or more years after the operation there is a 2 per cent chance of dislocation even with hips that have shown no evidence of any trouble. Why? Patients grow old, and muscles become weaker and stretch around the hip. Revision surgery is used to manage this problem.

A less likely complication is an infection many years after the original surgery. This can occur when another operation, for example dental surgery, releases bacteria in to your bloodstream and some establish themselves at the site of the prosthesis. Another source could be from urinary tract infection.

In time the femur and the acetabulum, which have been weakened because of hip replacement, could fracture. These bones can heal spontaneously, but they might need revision surgery.

Finally, some complications cannot be managed without risks greater than those surrounding the original surgery itself. The joint has to be saved by some radical means. One way is to remove the hip (called **excision arthroplasty**). This operation is done as a last resort. It is an old operation, from which patients recover with a surprising degree of mobility. About a quarter of the patients can walk without support afterwards, and about 80 per cent walk with a stick.

Revision surgery

Tess was the only informant who had revision surgery; Helen and Terri were subject to repeated operations for their rheumatoid arthritis.

Revision surgery does not enjoy the same rate of success as the original surgery. However, the success rate has improved in recent years. In many ways revision surgery is like the original, but there are some important differences from the patient's point of view. In the revision operation blood loss is greater, so more blood will be called for in your autologous blood donation.

Second, the surgeon must discover whether the hip is infected before operating. This is a difficult task. Special blood tests and scans are used; also an **aspiration** might be called for, a small operation in which a needle is put into the hip to sample fluid. If there is no infection the surgeon undertakes a one-stage operation, taking out the old hip and putting in another new one. If there is infection, the surgeon does the operation in two stages, taking out the infected hip, leaving the patient without a hip for six weeks or more, and, when the infection has been dealt with, inserting the new hip.

Revision surgery will take longer than the surgery for the original new hip. Your surgeon might have to work inside the pelvis rather than from the outside. The old prosthesis could be difficult to remove because it has got itself into an unexpected position. New bone-cutting techniques have been developed to overcome these difficulties, especially the problem of removing the old cement.

Cement-free prostheses are thought to be easier to revise and to give a better revision. Nevertheless, some surgeons will say that they too can be difficult to revise. The prevailing view is that a fully cemented prosthesis is suitable for older people with a life expectancy of ten years or less; cement-free implants are for people younger than 65.

For the revision operation, the question might arise: cemented or cementless hip? This is not always easily decided. As yet there is not enough evidence to conclude that results are improved with modern cementing techniques. Some surgeons prefer one to the other for different patients. This decision probably depends on how much bone has gone during the life of the implant. If the bone has to be rebuilt because of much bone loss, part of the patient's bone from elsewhere may be used, or perhaps, if a bone bank is available, bone will be taken from there. Some surgeons use artificial bone. Results from such operations are not easy to predict.

When the bone loss has been made up, the new prosthesis can be inserted. It might be a little longer and broader than the original implant, and it might be necessary to make a special fixture to secure the acetabulum.

With a revised hip, you will not be as mobile as before and will probably need crutches for longer. You might have to wear a hip brace to hold the new joint in place until your muscles heal. You will be in hospital a little longer; medical staff will be more concerned about the possibility of infection, and antibiotics will probably be used for a little longer.

How long will your new hip last?

For three reasons this question cannot be answered easily.

First, more than 90 per cent of new hips are satisfactory for several years after the operation. Later, satisfaction diminishes and the meaning of the word changes. A complete absence of discomfort for ten years could be satisfactory to some patients; the development of slight, erratic discomfort for a year or two after five years free of pain could be satisfactory for others. To settle the question of what 'satisfactory' means, it would be necessary to collect accurate records on all hip replacements so that your new hip and those of others could be monitored and assessed regularly. In Sweden a data bank of 150,000 records on hip replacement is kept, but complete and accurate records are not kept on a national basis in Australia, Britain or the USA. To answer this question, a clearing house of data on hip replacements is needed. It would need to expand constantly because the number of hip replacements is growing annually by many thousands a year, around the world.

Second, how and when do we assess the effectiveness of the operation? Do we ask how the patient feels? Do we look only at X-rays? After one, five, ten years? Looking at X-rays only would not be satisfactory because there is evidence that some X-rays indicate a technical failure in the new hip while the patient feels no discomfort at all.

Third, it is not usual for a reputable medical publication to present results of new hip replacements until at least five years after the follow-up data have been collected.

So the question is better put as: what affects the life of my hip? The experience of surgeons indicates that the younger the patient the shorter the hip life. If you are young, busy, active, and sporty, then your hip will probably wear out sooner than the hip of an older person who walks little and has a desk job. Ernst, who leads an active life, took the view that a new hip in his mid forties might be followed by revision surgery when he was 60. In the meantime he will had have much pleasure playing golf! Second, the more obese the patient, the shorter the hip life. So it seems that you can avoid or delay the need for revision surgery by watching your weight.

Use will affect the life of the new hip. The prosthesis wears, and it might loosen. The failure rate seems to double between ten and fifteen years after the operation. The femoral head lasts longer than the plastic part of the new acetabulum. It is not clear whether cemented or cementless hips last longer. After revision surgery, it seems that the second new hips do not last as long as the originals.

Also, the design of the new hip seems to affect its life. But the evidence for this is not sufficiently reliable.

To get as much life out of your new hip as you can, it appears that you should see the surgeon regularly, at least once every year after the first year. Also it is important to attend quickly to any infection, exercise regularly in a way that maintains the strength of your hip muscles and does not permit jarring of the new hip, keep your weight down, and avoid carrying very heavy objects and crossing your legs excessively.

9

Conclusions and recommendations

From patients' experiences in getting their new hip come advice and recommendations about five decisions. The decisions involve two feelings; one is based on ability to move, and the other on tolerance for pain. You will want a new hip when the pain is affecting your personal, family, and working life. You will need a new hip when the activities that you love are no longer possible.

Why can't you move? Why are you in so much pain? Everyone has their story. These stories provide intriguing personal information, but the technical reasons for pain and immobility come from doctors and medical specialists.

Eventually you will find that you must make several decisions about the pain and the inability to move. If the pain is crippling, the first decision is whether to accept surgery or find other treatments. A doctor can direct you to specialists in rheumatology and surgery for the information you will need to make this decision. A rheumatologist can advise you on the present state of your hip; an orthopaedic surgeon can guide you on the surgery for a new hip.

The surgeon expects you to ask questions. Your questions could be about: when and where to have a new hip; how to get yourself ready for the operation; taking up a special diet, possibly a weight loss program, exercises, and medications; blood transfusions and donations; the length of stay in hospital; pain following surgery; the site of the scar; stages of recovery; what can go wrong; limits to what you can do; when to go back to work; what sports you can play; the costs of hip replacement; getting your home ready for your recovery; legal consent to the operation; the risks of surgery; and precautions to take at home after the operation and for how long.

Surgeons want to be recognised for their work. They operate best with people who accept the role of patient, and follow them as the major adviser and central authority on new hips. If the surgeon leaves you with doubts, distress, and deep misgivings about how you and that surgeon might work together, see another surgeon. The choice of surgeon is the second decision, and, like the first, it is yours. Thereafter all vital decisions are your surgeon's.

Your third decision is to accept fully the role of patient. Patients, like surgeons and nurses, are expected to prepare for an operation. When you undergo surgery you suffer for a short period, recover gradually, and return to better health. This process is supervised by different medical staff. You might not accept this role fully or find ways to avoid it. If you feel suspicious, untrusting, and doubt the ability of people caring for you, your recovery will probably be joyless and distressing. Such patients tend to be childish and want to intrude on the treatment that they have agreed to accept. Doctors find them irritating, nurses have great difficulty wanting to care for them, and physiotherapists get annoyed. Consequently the success of the operation is impeded, and recovery is unsatisfactory to everyone. Becoming a competent patient requires work and the full acceptance of a short, necessary period of physical dependence on those who care for you.

Your fourth decision is to recognise the role allocated to you for recovery at home. When you get home, your rate of recovery might be held up by medical, physical, and personal problems.

Prominent medical problems are infection, blood clotting, and dislocation of the new hip. Speak with your surgeon if there is any evidence of infection, such as swelling of your legs, pain in the calf, red, hot, swelling around the surface of your wound, or a persistent rise in temperature. You should phone the surgeon if pain emerges in your chest or if you have problems breathing or coughing when you are at rest.

Finally, if you think you have dislocated your new hip, call the surgeon. The warning signs are a click or clunk in the new hip, sudden pain, and loss of control over your operated leg. It might also seem a little shorter and turn outward. Pain increases. Follow the surgeon's advice on whether to use a car or an ambulance to go to hospital.

Physical problems at home are legion, but most can be anticipated. To avoid falling, use non-skid, flat shoes; walk with a stick, crutches, or frame, and have chairs in place for you to rest. Tread carefully. Look out for hazards like slippery surfaces, loose rugs or carpets, spilled fluids, toys and reading material on the floor, boisterous children, and pets that dash and jump. So that you can reach without toppling, put items you need at waist height or slightly above.

When you travel far from home get a note from your doctor saying that you have a new metal hip. This could make you less of a hazard at airports and other security areas.

Exercise regularly, keep a pillow between your legs in bed, take your anticoagulants, adhere to the 90-degree rule, avoid crossing your legs, and do anything else your surgeon says.

Personal problems accompany you home from hospital. In hospital you were improving noticeably, but at home recovery becomes slow and uneven. You will get better and feel happier if you accept the bad days with the good. When you feel low, you will probably go a little further down than usual. Accept this feeling, and alert yourself to the positive: good things around you, new places you would like to walk to, and different activities you would like to do. When you feel high and believe your full recovery is only hours away, accept this too, then pace yourself.

As you recover you will find your lost sense of humour. Your carer will listen while you talk about how your feelings change; exercises and deep breathing will help you with those feelings.

These recommendations will help you to be a competent patient. As such you will conclude that you must be patient for the natural progress of recovery to catch up with what you demand.

The reward? Freedom from pain and ease of movement will give you a new life.

Glossary

abduction

The movement of one limb away from the midline of the body.

acetabulum, acetabula fossa, cotyloid cavity

Either of the two sockets, one on each side of the hip, into which the head of the femur fits. Together the acetabulum and the femur head make up your hip joint.

acupuncture

A Chinese treatment system in which thin metal needles are inserted into special spots beneath the skin to relieve symptoms. Some authorities assume that the needles help release endorphins, the brain's natural painkillers.

acute pain

Intense, severe pain that appears suddenly.

adduction

The movement of a limb towards the midline of the body.

anaesthetic

A means by which all sensation is abolished from the whole body (general anaesthetic) or a limited part of the body (local anaesthetic). With a general anaesthetic the patient loses consciousness of their body and surroundings because the activity of the **central nervous system** is depressed. *See also* epidural anaesthetic.

analgesic

A drug that relieves pain. Some analgesics are mild and recommended for headaches and toothaches, e.g. aspirin and paracetamol; other drugs are strong, e.g. pethidine and morphine, and are used to relieve the severe pain of surgery. The potent analgesics can lead to drug dependence, so they are only used when a doctor prescribes them.

angina

A sense of suffocation or suffocating pain.

anticoagulants

Drugs used to prevent the clotting of your blood. Heparin is a natural anticoagulant and is produced by the liver and in white blood cells, as well as other places, by preventing the final stages of blood clotting. A purified form is extracted and used in serious cases of blood clotting. Its main side effect is incessant bleeding. A synthetic anticoagulant is warfarin, which does not act as quickly as heparin. Either may be used to treat thrombosis (blood clotting) after surgery.

anti-inflammatories

Drugs that relieve the pain of inflamed joints. The most common anti-inflammatory drugs mentioned by my informants were Naprosyn, Indocid, and Voltaren. They are all prescription drugs of the NSAID (non-steroidal anti-inflammatory drug) group. Indocid is a trade name for indomethacin, an effective, long-used drug for many types of arthritis and the pain that accompanies inflammation of joints and soft tissues; also used for gout, bursitis, inflammation in and around tendons, and treatment of menstrual pain. It brings relief by inhibiting substances (prostaglandins) from acting on local tissues to produce inflammation. Its side effects are nausea, vomiting, sometimes diarrhoea, heartburn, headache, dizziness, light-headedness, and ulcers. Taken with aspirin or steroids it could lead to peptic ulcers and bleeding, and it might reduce the effect of blood pressure and fluid tablets. With alcohol it sometimes helps to irritate the stomach. Also it can interfere with blood clotting. Naprosyn and Naprosyn SR is the trade name for naproxen and is a drug similar to Indocid. It has much the same effects. Voltaren is the trade name for diclofenc. It has the same effects as the other two, although the side effects appear to be less frequent.

arthritis

The inflammation of one's joints indicated by swelling, warmth, redness of skin, pain, and restriction of movement. It appears in more than 200 forms, the most noted of which are osteoarthritis, rheumatoid arthritis, gout, and tuberculosis. The disease is found by examining the pattern of inflammation, X-rays, blood tests, and synovial fluid taken from between the affected joints. In the case of arthritis of the hip, the disease is caused most often by the degeneration of cartilage membrane between the femur and the acetabulum. It is treated with analgesics and anti-inflammatory drugs.

aspiration

If a new hip needs replacement, the surgeon might sample the hip joint to see whether there is any infection in the fluid at the site of the prosthesis. The same procedure is sometimes followed in the diagnosis of arthritis in the hip.

autologous blood donation/transfusion

A donation of your own blood to a blood bank, which in turn makes the blood available at the time of your operation. The procedure reduces the chances of infection. The term *autologous* means from oneself to oneself.

avascular necrosis

The death of the head of the femur caused by a lack of blood vessels at the site of the cartilage where the femur meets the acetabulum.

bed rashes

While you are in a hospital bed, heat rashes sometimes appear on the back or the buttocks. Often they are the result of using plastic liners in bed; also they might be due to drug allergies or reactions to an anaesthetic. Fungal rashes might be due to the failure to clear away soap when washing. Rashes can be treated with topical applications.

blood clot

A solid mass of protein in which blood cells are caught. The clot (or thrombus) appears in blood vessels, the heart or elsewhere as the result of blood coagulation. If it finds its way to the heart or lungs, it could be fatal. *See also* thrombosis.

blood count

The numbering of different blood cells in a known amount of blood. *See* haemoglobin.

bone bank

A deep freezer in which bone is kept for bone grafting.

calcification

A normal process in bone formation wherein calcium salts are deposited in tissue.

cardiovascular system

A vital system that includes the heart and two networks of blood vessels, the pulmonary and systemic circulation systems. Through the heart, lungs, and other vital organs blood is carried around the body, thereby transporting nutrients and oxygen to the tissues, and removing waste products.

cartilage

A grey to white, dense tissue that connects parts of the body. In adults it appears in three forms: between the joints it is hyaline cartilage; in tendons and invertebral discs it is fibrocartilage; in the external ear it is elastic cartilage.

CAT or CT scan

Computerised axial tomography, now known as computerised tomography, is used like an X-ray to provide images of structures deep in the body by bringing them into sharp focus and leaving selected others blurry.

catheter

A catheter is a flexible tube passed into the body to insert or remove fluid. In certain disorders a urinary catheter is passed into the bladder to empty it before an operation or to allow urine to be drained from the bladder after an operation. Some surgeons prefer not to use a catheter to avoid infection.

cemented, cementless or cement-free prosthesis

Prostheses at the hip joint might or might not be cemented in place. The decision is made by the surgeon. If cemented, the prosthesis is held in place in the femur and the acetabulum with a type of cement similar to that dentists use for our teeth. The layer between the prosthesis and the bone is the cement mantle. In the new hip the cementless or cement-free prosthesis is rough on the outside, and is held in place by the strength of the bone as it grows over the rough surface of the prosthesis and secures it to the leg.

central nervous system

The brain and the spinal cord, which together integrate the body's nervous activities.

Charnley pillow

An abduction pillow designed to ensure that the patient does not cross their legs while recovering from a hip replacement operation. The pillow is named after Sir John Charnley (1911–82), who first proposed that a new hip inserted into the patient be fixed to the bone with acrylic cement in 1959.

chronic pain

Pain that persists for a long time with little noticeable change, usually more than two or three months.

Clexane

A synthetic anticoaguiant drug. *See* warfarin.

contracture

Shrinking and shortening of muscles, without any increase in strength, which is usually the result of pain or disuse of muscle brought about by inflammation or injury. As the soft tissues around the joint contract, the joint can become deformed. In the hip the commonest contracture is the flexion contracture; the hip joint slowly flexes and ceases to straighten.

deep muscle fascia

The sheath around the muscle that borders on the prosthesis in the new hip.

deep vein thrombosis (DVT)

A cardiovascular complication in which blood clots establish themselves in the deep veins of the calf and thigh where they cannot be seen. After a hip operation DVT is thought to be preventable with the use of white stockings that go from hip to toe on both legs.

dislocation

Dislocation of the hip occurs usually with a clunking sound; it is followed by pain, which increases. You will be unable to turn your hip or move without added pain. Rarely can a hip dislocate painlessly. The hip can be replaced under an X-ray screen with traction or by some special manipulative technique. An anaesthetic could be used, depending on the amount of pain and the procedure employed. Treatment will be followed by a short period of bed rest, and later by normal walking with care not to dislocate again.

drip, intravenous

A tube for the continuous injection of blood, plasma, saline, glucose, or other fluid into a vein. The fluid is in a suspended bottle, and it drips down the tube to a hollow needle in the patient's vein, usually near the wrist.

embolism

Obstruction of an artery by a clot of blood, fat or air. Embolisms are usually treated with anticoagulants like heparin and warfarin.

endometriosis

A condition in which tissue similar to the lining of the uterus appears elsewhere in the pelvis, and complicates diagnosis and treatment of hip complaints.

endorphins

One of a group of chemical compounds that occur naturally in the brain and have pain-relieving properties.

epidural anaesthetic

An anaesthetic that involves an injection of an appropriate drug into the epidural space between the outermost surface of the spinal cord and vertebral canal. It is given when the patient is lying on one side. Usually it is given to bring pain relief during childbirth. It is recommended for new hip operations when, in the anaesthetist's and the surgeon's opinion, it is appropriate to reduce the requirements for general anaesthetic drugs. Under the direction of an anaesthetist you are given injections and if necessary gases to inhale, and as a result you are not conscious of surgery or the conditions under which it is carried out.

epiphysial dysplasia

Abnormal development of the end of a long bone.

excision athroplasty

An old operation, done only as a last resort, in which a joint is removed. Almost 25 per cent of patients whose hip is removed can still walk afterwards.

extension

Stretching and straightening your hip so that you can bend your leg backwards.

extension arm, extension hand, pick-up stick, hand reacher

A most useful device to help you pick up things without bending or reaching for them.

femur

The long thigh bone, which goes from pelvis to knee. Its head fits into the acetabulum to make the moving part of the hip joint. If the growth area at the upper end of the bone becomes deformed, the head of the femur can degenerate and the hip joint can become inflamed; in serious cases it must be replaced with a prosthesis.

flexion

Bending of a joint so that the bones that form it are brought closer, e.g. in the case of your hip, when you bend it so that your knee is closer to your chin.

flexion contracture

The most common contracture of the hip when it is in trouble; the hip flexes slowly and in time no longer straightens. This makes for limping, and over time walking becomes difficult. Eventually you might decide that you need a new hip.

gout

Inflammation around the foot, ankle, and sometimes the knee. The area becomes red and painful to the touch. Uric acid and its salts accumulate in the bloodstream and at the joints. It can lead to acute gouty arthritis and chronic destruction of the joints.

haemochromatosis

A hereditary blood disorder in which the body excessively absorbs and retains iron. It is evident in the bronze and greyish colour of the skin. The disorder impairs the normal functioning of many organs, thus making it necessary to draw off blood regularly, or to administer a drug that leads the iron to be excreted.

haemoglobin

A substance in red blood cells that combines with oxygen, and is the means by which oxygen is carried through the body. Haemoglobin takes oxygen as blood passes through the lungs and releases it as the blood passes through the tissues of the body. Normally blood contains 12–18 units of haemoglobin. In hospital blood samples are taken, the number of units in the blood is measured in a blood count, and the extent to which oxygen is getting to the tissues is estimated. If the estimate is too low, the level of oxygen in the blood might be inadequate, recovery from surgery could be impeded, and a blood transfusion could be called for.

hand reacher

See extension arm.

heparin

See anticoagulants.

heterotopic ossification

Heterotopic (or ectopic) ossification is the formation of small pieces of bone in places where it is not normally expected, as in the soft tissues around the new hip after the operation. Usually it causes no personal problems, and appears as small unrelated blobs of bone in unusual places. Nevertheless, the ossification (bone formation) can spread, and if it emerges in the space between the new ball and socket of the hip, and takes hold, the process is hard to correct. In extreme cases it can stop all movement of the new hip.

homoeopathy

A theory of medicine that assumes like cures like. It was devised by Samuel Hahnemann (1755–1843) in the late eighteenth century. Today it is an accepted form of alternative medicine followed by a few doctors. Patients are given tiny quantities of a drug that is able to produce the disorder from which the patient is assumed to suffer.

hypnosis

A procedure for helping or inducing a person who is receptive to suggestion to take part in the treatment of their disorder, e.g. as a cure for addiction and in other forms of psychotherapy.

Independent Living Centre

A place where you can see all the items that help a disabled person to live independently. A visit to such a centre would help you plan your rehabilitation and what you might need to make your recovery less of an effort.

infection

Infection, a serious complication that might arise from surgery, occurs when the body is invaded by some harmful organisms. Common organisms are bacteria, fungi, and viruses. They can be transmitted from people, animals, insects, soil, and in many other ways to a person. Treatment with drugs is usually effective, but not for common viral infections like colds and influenza. The common symptoms are pain, swelling, inflammation, and red and hot skin.

insomnia

The inability to fall asleep, or sleep long enough so that one does not wake feeling weary. With insomnia, people feel tired all the time. The cause is not easily identified; nevertheless disease, pain, and worry are commonly thought to be reasons for the disorder.

iron tablets

Iron tablets are taken for a week before the operation to supplement the blood with iron lost in making autologous blood donations.

Moore's prosthesis

An early treatment of hip disorder in which only part of the hip, the head of the femur, is replaced as a treatment for arthritis. Today the procedure is sometimes used for treating some patients with a fractured hip.

morphine

A potent analgesic and narcotic drug to relieve pain and induce sleep. It is taken orally or by injection, and sometimes produces nausea, loss of appetite, confusion, and constipation. It makes you feel euphoric, and it can become addictive.

narcotics

Drugs that induce stupor and insensibility and relieve pain. The most common is morphine, a derivative of opium. The term is also used to refer to drugs used in a general anaesthetic. Because morphine is addictive it is rarely used as a sleep-inducing drug. It is still used to relieve severe pain.

nausea

The feeling that one is about to vomit.

NSAIDs

See anti-inflammatories.

occupational therapy/therapist

In the treatment of physical and psychiatric cases activities are planned to make greatest use of a patient's capabilities, depending on their needs. The occupational therapy centres on activities such as woodwork, metalwork, art, pottery, social skills for psychiatric cases, and leisure activities for geriatric patients. Such therapists are skilled in analysing home situations in which patients live while recovering from surgery.

orthopaedic surgeon

A surgeon who corrects deformities due to damage and disease to the bones and their joints. A highly specialised branch of surgery, orthopaedics involves operations, traction, manipulation, the use of surgical devices to support unstable bones, and prostheses.

orthotic

A surgical appliance to help weakened joints.

ossification

The formation of bone.

osteoarthritis, primary and secondary

Primary osteoarthritis is a disease of the joint cartilage; associated with it are changes in the bones at the joint, which wear and become painful and unable to operate easily. The disease occurs primarily in hips, knees, and thumbs. It can be caused by a trauma as well as by gradual wear and tear; it is more common among those past middle age; it can complicate diseases of other joints, as in rheumatoid arthritis (secondary arthritis). Osteoarthritis is observed in X-rays where the cartilage in the joint space has been lost and the area between the two bones is so narrow as to be non-existent. The disease is treated with aspirin and other analgesics, reducing weight on the joint with weight loss and a walking stick, and corrective surgery as in total hip or knee replacement.

osteolysis

Inflammation, dissolution and loss of bone usually through disease. It can occur around the operated area years after a hip replacement due to small pieces of debris appearing as the new hip wears and loosens.

osteopathy

The diagnosis and treatment of bone and joint diseases based on the belief that much of the trouble is related to disorders of the musculo-skeletal system. Back pain is much relieved by such treatment.

osteoporosis

The loss of bony tissue that leads to bones becoming thin, weak, and brittle. It is common among elderly people, and women past menopause.

osteotomy

A surgeon's term to indicate a division of the bone such that the bone is cut and rejoined at a different angle. The operation reduces the pain and disability associated with arthritis.

Panadeine Forte

A strong painkiller with codeine.

paracetamol

A mild painkiller for headache, toothache, and rheumatism.

pathologist

A doctor who specialises in diseases. A pathologist observes blood, urine, faeces, and diseased tissue, and uses X-rays and other techniques to study diseases in an effort to understand their causes.

patient-controlled analgesia (PCA)

In some hospitals patients may control their own painkiller under close supervision of the medical staff. With this system it is not possible for the patient to overdose.

pelvis

The bony structure around the lower part of the trunk, which protects the organs of the lower abdomen and is attached to the bones and muscles of the lower limbs.

pethidine

A strong analgesic that induces sleep and relieves severe pain. It is taken orally or by injection. Its side effects include nausea, dizziness, dry mouth, hallucinations, and it can become addictive.

physiotherapist

A person trained in physiotherapy, the branch of treatment that uses physical procedures to promote healing. Physiotherapists use light, infra-red and ultraviolet rays, heat, electric current, hydrotherapy, manipulation, massage, stretching, and exercises.

pick-up stick

See extension arm.

prosthesis

An artificial part attached to or implanted in your body.

pulmonary embolus or embolism

A clot of blood that moves from your leg to your lungs and obstructs the pulmonary artery. If it is large it can produce heart failure and sudden death. Chest discomfort, shortness of breath, and chest pain when inhaling indicate the possibility of this dangerous disorder. Minor pulmonary emboli are treated with anticoagulant drugs heparin or warfarin. A major pulmonary embolism can require surgery or the infusion of a special enzyme.

radiologist

A paramedical specialist who uses radiation such as X-rays and radioactive substances to diagnose and treat disease.

reaming

Widening a hole with a borer; the means by which the surgeon removes bone so that parts of the prosthesis can be fitted into the femur or the acetabulum.

rehabilitation centre

A hospital-like place where ill or injured patients go to be restored to normal health, or to prevent a disability from getting worse.

revision surgery, revision replacement

Surgery for the replacement of a new hip. Such surgery is more complicated than the original operation for a new hip, and requires a longer period of recovery.

rheumatoid arthritis

The second most common arthritic disease after osteoarthritis. It involves joints of the wrists, fingers, feet, ankles, hips, knees, and shoulders. The joints are affected symmetrically. The effects can be extremely severe or rather mild. Diagnosis is by blood analysis and from X-rays. Although the disease can resolve itself spontaneously, eventually there is a relapse, and the patient becomes progressively worse. Treatment involves anti-inflammatory drugs and hip replacement.

rheumatologist

A doctor who specialises in disease of the joints, tendons, muscles, ligaments, and associated parts of the body.

sciatic nerve

The sciatic nerve is the thickest nerve in the body. It runs down the back, around the buttocks, and down the side of the leg. Above the knee joint it divides and proceeds in two branches to the muscles and skin of the lower leg. If pinched, irritated, compressed or otherwise put under pressure, it hurts and produces sciatica.

sciatica

A pain down the back and along the outer side of the thigh into the leg and foot. Usually the cause is a degenerating disc between vertebrae, which protrudes and presses on the thick sciatic nerve. The pain comes suddenly, sometimes after twisting or lifting something heavy. The leg becomes numb and weak. Treatment is bedrest, and perhaps surgery if bedrest fails.

spinal anaesthetic

See anaesthetic and epidural anaesthetic.

spondylitis

Inflammation of the synovial joints of the backbone.

suppository

A medical preparation in solid form placed in the rectum or vagina. Rectal suppositories contain lubricants to free the rectum, drugs that act locally, or drugs that act elsewhere in the body.

synovial fluid

The thick and colourless fluid that lubricates the joints and tendon sheaths. In the hip joint it lubricates the acetabulum and femur head, and makes it possible for them to articulate a hip joint that operates freely.

synovium

The lining of a joint, which encourages the absorption and the production of synovial fluid, which makes the joint move easily.

TED/DVT stockings

Thromboembolic deterrent or deep vein thrombosis white stockings, which help prevent embolisms forming and going to your lungs or heart where they could be fatal. Stockings reach from waist to toe.

thrombosis

A condition whereby blood changes from being liquid to solid. *See also* blood clot.

Urecoline

A drug, bethanchol chloride, used to help a patient suffering from urinary retention after an operation. It is given by injection or tablets.

urinary retention

The state of being unable to urinate, largely due to the shock of the operation to vital organs around the hip. A urinary catheter can be used to relieve this condition.

vegan

A person who does not eat or use animal products.

warfarin

A synthetic anticoagulant drug with the trade names Coumadin and Marevan. It is often prescribed for some weeks after a hip operation to thin the blood and lessen the chances of a pulmonary embolism.

Informants

Bernard, in his fifties, drives the school bus in a small country town. His brother had a new hip, but felt it was not as successful as he had hoped. Nevertheless, Bernard looked into the possibility of having a similar operation because he had the same pain as his brother. After seeing a surgeon at the large suburban hospital where his brother had been, Bernard decided to have the operation. He felt anxious about the anaesthetic but was assured that it would be no trouble and underwent surgery. He felt that he was nursed very well, and recovered from the experience cheerfully. Now he is driving the school bus again, and is free of pain.

Betty, a widow, is in her eighties and lives alone in an apartment with thirty-two steps to its entrance. She travels frequently to Europe. A student of languages, she became fluent in German and for many years taught in high school. Born with one leg slightly shorter than the other, she wears an orthotic. She lived a life free of pain until one day her back froze while she was cleaning her home. In time the problem was traced to her hip. Since her hip operation she has been comfortable, and was especially pleased that the surgeon was able to lengthen her operated leg. After the operation she invented useful aids to make recovery easier at home.

Charles is in his sixties and was in politics for many years. As a young man he loved exercise and sport, and today feels that too much thumping around the running track and the tennis and squash courts was responsible for his hip trouble. In hospital he cheerfully entered into an agreement with the surgeon to be a subject for a study of the relative effectiveness of anticoagulants used after the hip operation. Because he was in politics so long he appreciated the current financial and medical problems of hospitals. His recovery was longer than that of most other informants. Now he feels healthy, writes for newspapers, and is a university scholar.

Doug is in his fifties and works as a university architect supervising building construction. When he was about 50 he found that the pain in his knee and unexpected wastage in his leg were not easy to explain because he was an inveterate bike rider and played much sport. He thought that his slight cerebral palsy might have hindered his movements. When he found that his hip was in trouble, he arranged to wait a year before having surgery. The pain became difficult to bear towards the end of that time. In hospital he had a distressing complication after the operation, but recovered quickly. When he came home he exercised assiduously and, with the help of hydrotherapy, recovered well.

Ernst is a psychiatrist and an athlete. He suffered a congenital hip disorder. Nevertheless, as a young man he trained for the Olympics and made the team. In his mid forties he decided to have two new hips, and studied the medical literature closely to prepare for the operation, which would be done by a colleague who was also a close friend. Because he was so fit Ernst recovered from both operations quickly, and now moves as if he had never been incapacitated by hip trouble.

Fred is in his early seventies and was a prominent social scientist who years ago worked in hospitals. When he learned he needed a new hip he investigated the operation, studied the medical literature, was dubious about the surgery, and concluded that he would wait for surgical procedures to improve. He had difficulty finding the kind of surgeon he wanted. He chose to be operated on at a public hospital, and was not happy with some aspects of the nursing he received. After the operation he became ill while recovering at home and had to go back to hospital to have a blood clot treated. Today he is well, plays golf, and enjoys his new occupation — painting pictures and studying art.

Helen is in her late twenties and studies at university. She has rheumatoid arthritis, which was not diagnosed early. Her mother, an anthropologist, battled to get her daughter the best medical advice. Helen has had many operations on her fragile hips. She walks with underarm crutches. She became a vegetarian, and used her experiences in hospital to study first hand how a hospital staff catered for a young patient with special dietary needs. She has a remarkably cheerful attitude to her serious complaint, and seems determined to live as well as she can with it.

Mario, in his late fifties, runs a small business in the country. He and his wife specialise in Italian cooking at their roadside restaurant close to a wine-growing district. Mario travels the district encouraging the development of his business, and supplies fine foods and wines for shops and restaurants like the one his family has. His hip trouble was partly related to a blood disorder — too much iron in the blood — and he was pleased to find a surgeon who was an expert in both problems. At the time he spoke about his experiences he believed that a second hip would not be needed. However, he recently had surgery on the other hip and now has two new hips.

Nell is middle-aged, lives alone, and works part-time. Her arthritis limited her movements moderately until, on returning from a trip overseas, her hip began giving her much pain, and she found that she needed a walking stick. She had difficulty finding a surgeon she liked, and felt that her recovery was a little slower than that of most others. After hospital she went to a rehabilitation centre, learned much to help her at home, and recovered gradually by going for long walks in the neighbourhood.

Sonomi is a busy director of a city art gallery that regularly changes its exhibitions and thrives on a high reputation. She chose her surgeon carefully and was most concerned about her anaesthetist's procedures. Her operation was successful, and she went to a rehabilitation centre, where she learned little that was relevant to her activities at home but benefited from hydrotherapy. Because she was so involved in her gallery work, and so keen to return to her administrative duties, she felt restless about her rate of recovery while at home. Now she is back at work, and enjoys it more because the pain has gone and she can move easily.

Terri is in her thirties and has had rheumatoid arthritis since she was 15. She had traces of it earlier, but did not realise then what it was. The disease advanced quickly. She had many operations to relieve the suffering, spent long periods in hospital, used many different techniques to arrest the spread of the disease — including fasting — and put every effort into enjoying what she can from life. She is determined to make the best of her life; she became a university student, travelled, looks after her home above a bookstore, helps her husband in the shop, and in many other ways assumes the life of a person without a serious and lasting illness. She insists that those who care for suffers like herself, especially friends and family members, be recognised for their efforts and compassion.

Tess is in her eighties. She had three operations on the same hip. As a young woman she had been a theatre nurse, was familiar with the procedures of surgeons, and thought surgery was excellent for relief of suffering. She felt her first hip replacement was successful until eight years later when her hip implant loosened. The revision operation seemed successful, but discomfort in her leg arose and could not be banished with physiotherapy. The third operation brought little relief, and her leg is weak. Today she feels disappointed about the lack of improvement in her operated leg, but has accepted the limitation on her movements and works around it.

Wendy was injured by a truck when she was a girl. At the time modern hip replacement surgery was in its infancy, and she was too young for a total hip replacement. She had to wait until middle age before she could contemplate a new hip. In the meantime she became a nurse, married, and had five children. By the time her children had grown up she was advised that hip surgery was well enough advanced for her to have the operation. Like others, she felt anxious about modern anaesthetic techniques, but was assured that all would be well. She now moves around easily and without pain.

Selected reading

Bower, R., Kerschbaumer, F. and Poisel, S. (eds). 1996. *Atlas of Hip Surgery.* New York: Thieme. A book for those who need to see the technical details of hip surgery as it is performed.

Cowley, D.E. (1994). *Prosthesis for Total Hip Replacement.* Australian Institute of Health and Welfare: Health Care Technology Series No. 12. Canberra, ACT: Australian Government Publishing Service. A most informative research report to government on the cost and effectiveness of total hip replacement in Australia and evaluation of research on the subject.

Macnicol, M.F. (1995). *Colour Atlas of Osteotomy of the Hip.* London: Times Mirror. Mosby Year Book. A book for people who want to see details of the hip operation as it is performed.

McCullen, Geoffrey and Miller, Ryle jnr (1996). *Hip and Knee Replacement: A Patient's Guide.* New York: Norton. A useful clinical guide to hip and knee replacement.

National Institute of Health (1994). *Total Hip Replacement: National Institutes of Health Consensus Statement.* September 12–14. 12(5) No. 98. 1–31. Bethesda, Maryland: NIH Office of Medical Applications of Research. The most recent full report for doctors on research on hip replacement in the USA.

Pellicic, Paul and Padgett, Douglas E. (1995). *Atlas of Total Hip Replacement.* New York: Churchill Livingstone (Longman). A book for people who need a technical description of a hip operation as it is being done.

Pfitzner, Max C. (1991). *Hip Replacement: Care and Management.* Adelaide, SA: Desktop Publishing by Graphex. A full account of hip replacement for those who treat patients after the hip operation or who are in training, e.g. physiotherapists, nurses, and occupational therapists.

Ragg, Mark (1995). *So You're Having Hip Replacement.* Woollahra, NSW: Gore & Osment. An medical journalist's account of the basics of hip replacement, which helps individuals with hip trouble to decide whether a replacement would suit them. The book centres on what to expect from medical advisers, and give details of technical aspects of their work.

Star, Leonie (1993). *Hip Replacement: A Consumer's Guide.* Annandale, NSW: Federation Press. An encouraging account by a patient on her experiences when she had her hips replaced in 1991 and 1993. The author aims to inform, reduce anxiety, and support attempts by patients to understand what they can do about getting hips replaced. The author claims no knowledge of the practice of medicine.

Villar, Richard (1995). *Hip Replacement: A Patient's Guide to Surgery and Recovery.* London: Thorsons-HarperCollins. An account of hip surgery from a British doctor's viewpoint with comprehensive recommendations for recovery and an informative account of the history of the surgeon's work since the late 1940s.

Index